Core Clinical Skills for OSCEs in Medicine

To our students, who make it all worthwhile

Commissioning Editor: Laurence Hunter
Project Development Manager: Janice Urquhart
Project Manager: Nancy Arnott
Design direction: Judith Wright
Illustrated by: Robert Britton

Core Clinical Skills for OSCEs in Medicine

Tim Dornan MA BM BCh DM FRCP
Hospital Dean, Honorary Clinical Senior Lecturer and Consultant Physician,
Hope Hospital, Salford, Manchester, UK

Paul O'Neill MB ChB BSc(Hons) MD FRCP
Associate Dean for Medical Undergraduate Studies, Senior Lecturer and
Honorary Consultant in Geriatric Medicine, University of Manchester,
Manchester, UK

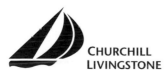

CHURCHILL
LIVINGSTONE

EDINBURGH LONDON NEW YORK PHILADELPHIA ST LOUIS SYDNEY TORONTO 2000

CHURCHILL LIVINGSTONE
An imprint of Harcourt Publishers Limited

© Harcourt Publishers Limited 2000

⮡ is a registered trademark of Harcourt Publishers Limited

The rights of Tim Dornan and Paul O'Neill to be identified as authors of this
work has been asserted by them in accordance with the Copyright, Designs
and Patents Act 1988.

First published 2000
 Reprinted 2001 (twice)

ISBN 0 443 06366 4

British Library Cataloguing in Publication Data
A catalogue record for this book is available from the British Library.

Library of Congress Cataloging in Publication Data
A catalog record for this book is available from the Library of Congress.

Note
Medical knowledge is constantly changing. As new information becomes
available, changes in treatment, procedures, equipment and the use of drugs
become necessary. The authors and the publishers have, as far as it is possible,
taken care to ensure that the information given in this text is accurate and up
to date. However, readers are strongly advised to confirm that the
information, especially with regard to drug usage, complies with latest
legislation and standards of practice.

The
publisher's
policy is to use
**paper manufactured
from sustainable forests**

Printed in China by RDC Group Limited
P/03

Up and down the land, medical education is undergoing change. Sparked off by 'Tomorrow's Doctors', the UK General Medical Council's radical manifesto for change, medical schools are revising their undergraduate curricula. There are even changes planned for Royal College examinations arising from a growing awareness that all is not well with the traditional long and short case examination format. What lies at the heart of this change is a realisation that medical education has tended to place too great an emphasis on factual *knowledge* – enter *skills* and *attitudes* – and that many examinations are unreliable and test the wrong things – enter the 'OSCE' (Objective Structured Clinical Examination).

We were stimulated to write, not by a blind devotion to the OSCE format, but by a wish to make our graduates confident that they are 'fit for purpose'. Our experience of making radical curriculum change in Manchester is that this can be achieved. First, teachers need to see medical competence as the goal of training and decide what knowledge, skills and attitudes their graduates must acquire. Next, they must make those educational objectives clear to their students. Then they must use appropriate educational methods to help students acquire them. Finally, they must assess students, and give them feedback on their performance. It seems a truism to say that the objectives of assessments should be determined by the objectives of the curriculum, and that assessments should be valid and reliable, but how many schools can actually describe their assessments in those terms?

When our students volunteered to take part in our first pilot OSCE examination some years ago, one of our senior professors commented that it was like 'turkeys voting for Christmas'. Since then, the biannual OSCEs have consistently had the thumbs-up from our students as relevant, fair, challenging and – dare one say it – even fun, in a kind of way. Examiners are less sure about the fun, but volunteer to take part and tolerate the repetitive nature of the task with good grace because they see value in it.

What we have done in this book is compile a set of medical tasks that are performed in one guise or another by every newly qualified doctor. We have tried to define within those tasks the *skills* that must be acquired to perform them. We have explained the skills, and described how they might be measured. We have lavished on our readers suggestions about how they might acquire the skills and polish them up so that they excel in examinations. We do so confident in the belief the 'cramming' for an OSCE examination will help build clinical competence, and that success in the exam will build well-founded confidence.

Although the short station undergraduate OSCE exam is the main focus of the book, we have strayed into long cases, short cases, other new types of examination such as the 'OSLER' and workplace clinical learning. We believe that the book will be of use to students in traditional curricula and facing traditional exams, as well as those confronted by the newer educational methods. Indeed, we hope that the book would be of use to a student facing no examinations at all! We hope that our thoughts may be of value to teachers who have to set OSCE exams. We also have one eye on the likely move towards OSCEs in postgraduate examinations and hope the book might be of some value to candidates and examiners.

We would not pick a fight with a student or teacher who dismissed OSCEs as a fad promoted by educationalists with nothing better to do. We would, however, defy anyone to argue that our trainees do not need to be supplied with the components of medical competence, and a workshop manual to assemble them, so that they are roadworthy when they qualify. If you, our reader, are more confident in your clinical skills when you have read the book, then the midnight oil we burned on it has not been wasted. Read on!

Tim Dornan   2000
Paul O'Neill   Manchester

Acknowledgements

We thank Neil Maredia, Liam Hosie, Chloe Baxter and Mark Dornan who read our early drafts and gave us 'the student view' and lots of valuable encouragement; Corinne Siddall, Paul Chadwick, Gordon Armstrong, Jackie Leigh, Sarah Smith and John Houghton who helped us with some details; and Laurence Hunter of Churchill Livingstone, who put us up to it in the first place!

Contents

OSCEs by system

 CARDIOVASCULAR

 **RESPIRATORY**

GASTROINTESTINAL

GENITOURINARY

NEUROLOGICAL

 **HAEMATOLOGICAL**

ENDOCRINE/METABOLIC

LOCOMOTOR

 INFECTIOUS DISEASES

 GENERAL

CHAPTER 1

Introduction

PREPARING FOR THE BIG DAY

You have probably bought this book because you are facing an OSCE examination. To help you prepare, our primary aims are to:

- Explain what an OSCE is
- Describe what format it might take
- Give you examples of typical stations
- Demonstrate how you might handle them, and what an examiner might be looking for
- Give you hints on how to develop your skills and prepare for the exam
- Present the material of the book in a way that helps you revise
- Give you ways of constructing complete 'exams' at different levels to judge your progress.

WORKING TOWARDS BASIC CLINICAL COMPETENCE

It would be an awful waste of energy if examinations – and the preparation that you put into them – were just an obstacle course. Exams are there to give you an incentive to become competent, and to give you (as well as your examiners and future patients) an assessment of just how competent you are. Clinical competence is an amalgam of knowledge, skills and attitudes. In writing this book, we also set out to write a 'primer' of basic clinical skills. To be more specific, we aimed to:

- Define a set of core skills
- Analyse and define the skills in a way that helps you perform them well
- Discuss some of the knowledge and attitudes related to those skills
- Define how you and your peers – as well as your future examiners – could measure performance of those skills.

Rather than cramming at the last minute, we advise you to take a far-sighted view of the OSCE. Build skills throughout your training. That way, you will see your confidence and competence grow and you will take exams in your stride.

THE OSCE

What is an OSCE?

An OSCE is an Objective Structured Clinical Examination. It was originally designed to reduce some of the problems associated with traditional clinical exams (i.e. 'long and short cases'). In an ideal assessment, all the variability in scores would come from the difference in performance/competence of the students being tested. Unfortunately, much of the variability in clinical examinations comes from the examiners taking candidates to see patients with different problems and asking them to do different things. Examiners also vary in how they mark students ('hawks and doves') so if you only see a pair of 'hawks', you may fail when your friend passes because she sees the examiners who never fail anybody. The OSCE increases the fairness of an exam by:

- Increasing the range of skills on which you are tested
- Increasing the number of examiners by whom you are assessed
- Marking against explicit criteria.

Standardised patients, volunteers and anatomical models

One way in which OSCEs differ from traditional long and short case examinations is in the use of simulation. In other words, the exam often tests a student in a 'laboratory' context, rather than at the bedside with a real patient. So, for example, a junior student may be asked to show to an examiner that he can go competently through the motions of examining the abdomen of a healthy volunteer without being expected to pick up abnormal signs. Thus a wide range of skills can be tested without having to recruit patients with specific diseases, and basic procedural competence is tested independently of (and usually at an earlier stage than) competence to detect abnormalities. Simulation allows skills to be tested that could not be tested on either volunteers or patients. Thus, rectal examination, vaginal examination or testicular examination are tested on anatomical models. The use of 'standardised patients' (volunteers who are trained to take on roles) extends simulation to history and communication skills. In many of the stations in this book, students are asked to take a history, or explain something to a standardised patient. A student may also be asked to break bad news or handle a more difficult problem of interpersonal communication with an actor or other person trained to simulate such situations. In preparing for an OSCE, remember that the emphasis is on simulation and on testing basic procedural competence in junior examinations. Remember, also, that nobody can be proven fit to qualify as a doctor by simulation alone so senior examinations will undoubtedly test competence with 'real' patients with 'real' symptoms and signs.

What form does a typical OSCE take?

Usually, students rotate around a 'circus' consisting of a number of 'stations' lasting a short, fixed time. In that way, all students are asked the same questions at identical stations. The exam often has between 10 and 20 stations, each lasting about 5 minutes. Thus 10–20 students can be examined in one 'round' of the circus in an exam lasting 50–100 minutes. An example of an OSCE for a junior clinical student is shown in Table 1.1. You might start anywhere from station 1 to station 16 and then rotate round to the next station each time the bell (alarm) sounds until you have finished all the stations.

What is being tested?

Different medical schools have different ideas about the purpose of an OSCE. Some see it mainly as a *knowledge test* (which makes it little different from an MCQ or viva). Others see it very much as a *skills test*, because that allows the OSCE to test students in a way that other types of assessment do not. We are firmly in the skills camp, the more so because it has allowed us to offer information

Table 1.1 A specimen OSCE at the end of junior clerkships

Station No.[1]	Title	Type of station	Length (minutes)	Brief description	System	Page no.
1	Chest pain	History	5	Take a history from a standardised patient	CVS	26
2	Present the history of chest pain	History	5	Present the history to an examiner; answer questions about heart disease	CVS	31
3	Respiratory examination 1	Examination	5	Demonstrate the skill on a volunteer	RS	89
4	Explain 24-h urine collection	Communication	5	Explain the procedure to a volunteer; answer questions about investigation of hypertension	GUS	262
5	Blood count	Interpretation	5	Interpret a lab slip; answer questions about possible causes of the abnormalities	Haem	174
6	Rest station	–	5	This gives you a little time to calm down and gather your wits	–	–
7	Measure blood pressure	Examination	5	Measure blood pressure on an electronic mannequin arm, which allows the examiner to test your accuracy	CVS	79
8	Basic life support	Procedure	5	Demonstrate the skill on a resuscitation dummy	General	224
9	Pyrexia	History	5	The examiner tests your knowledge of a history-taking skill in 'structured oral' format	General	65
10	Lumbar puncture	Communication	5	Interview a standardised patient to obtain informed consent; show awareness of the ethics of consent and knowledge of meningitis	Neurological	265

Table 1.1 *(cont'd)*

Station No.[1]	Title	Type of station	Length (minutes)	Brief description	System	Page no.
11	Venepuncture	Procedure	5	Perform venepuncture on an anatomical arm; answer questions about safe handling of specimens	General	227
12	Rest station	–	5	–	–	–
13	Rectal examination	Examination	5	Demonstrate the skill on an anatomical model and answer questions about diseases that might be found	GIS	101
14	Urea and electrolytes	Interpretation	5	The examiner shows you data, asks your interpretation, and then gives you further, increasingly complex, data to interpret	Cardiovascular	161
15	Examine vision	Examination	5	Demonstrate eye examination on a volunteer	Neurological	109
16	Record an ECG	Procedure	5	Demonstrate the skill on a volunteer, then interpret an ECG	Cardiovascular	190

[1]The 16 stations are arranged in a 'circus'. Sixteen students start simultaneously and rotate around the stations. You could enter the circus at any one of the 16 stations.

in this book which conventional textbooks do not. You would be well advised to find out as much as you can about the purpose and format of the OSCE you are facing. You may even find major differences between different OSCEs in the same medical school.

Note the mixture of skills in Table 1.1. These can be divided broadly into:

- Obtaining and presenting a **history** (Chapter 3). This may be with a volunteer ('standardised patient') or a 'real' patient.
- Physical **examination** (Chapter 4), which can involve demonstrating your skills on a patient (usually in a more senior examination), a normal volunteer or a mannequin (dummy).
- **Interpretation** skills (Chapter 5); applying your knowledge to clinical findings, data, radiographs, ECGs etc.
- **Procedure** skills (Chapter 6); often using mannequins.
- **Communication** skills (Chapter 7). Interpersonal communication other than history taking. This is likely to involve a standardised patient (see page 3).
- **Attitude** stations (Chapter 8); a short oral examination in which the examiner will probe your attitudinal approach to a particular situation (e.g. involving confidentiality of information). Table 1.1 does not have a station devoted to attitudes because it is pitched at the basic/intermediate level and complex attitudinal issues are more likely to be tested in senior exams.

What are examiners looking for?

Competence! In other words, a fluent demonstration of a skill, and the knowledge and attitudes associated with it. Marks will be awarded for:

- A confident approach
- A pace which indicates that you have taken trouble to acquire and consolidate the skill
- Dexterity in performing manual skills
- Good **applied** knowledge (purely abstract knowledge is of little clinical use). That must include knowledge of normal form and function as well as knowledge of disease
- Comprehensive, clear and considered answers showing that you have thought about the topic before and are not just 'fire-fighting'
- Level-headedness, even when the going is tough. For example, admitting that you do not know something rather than waffling
- Good communication with both the patient (volunteer) and examiner. That is important for two reasons:
  - Communication is **the** central clinical skill
  - Communication is the medium through which your attitudes will be tested.

How are OSCEs marked?

Figure 1.1 shows a specimen check-list for a basic OSCE station. You will see that marks are given for aspects of communication as well as the physical examination,

Examination 16: Neurological examination legs (motor)

Please assess the candidate's examination technique using the following criteria:

	Yes	No
1. Did the candidate clearly explain what examination they wanted to do?	—	—
2. Did the candidate give clear instructions about what they needed the patient to do during the examination (e.g. in testing power)?	—	—

	Not done 0 Marks	Inadequate 1 Mark	Adequate 2 Marks
3. Did you observe the candidate inspecting the legs?	—	—	—
4. Did the candidate compare the two sides during the examination?	—	—	—
5. Could the candidate elicit the quadriceps reflexes?	—	—	—
6. Could the candidate elicit the ankle reflexes?	—	—	—
7. Could the candidate elicit the plantar reflexes?	—	—	—
8. Was tone examined adequately?	—	—	—
9. Was clonus examined for?	—	—	—
10. Was power tested across all the joints?	—	—	—

Marks /18
Overall excellence /4
Total marks /22

General comments:

Figure 1.1 A specimen marking schedule

and that the examiner is given discretion to award marks for overall excellence. Note how your response to an instruction like *'Please examine motor function in this patient's legs'* is broken down into its component parts and marks are awarded on a three-point scale. See how much better you will do if you have learned the skill systematically and thoroughly than if you approach it in a haphazard way. In a number of the stations in this book, we show how candidates may be 'extended' from the basic skill to a more complex one, or into a related area of knowledge. If you want to get good marks in OSCEs:

- Don't just learn the basic skill, learn **around the skill** as well
- Don't just learn abstract theoretical knowledge, **apply** your knowledge
- Take as many opportunities as possible to practise your skills and receive feedback from a teacher.

Common mistakes in OSCEs

We give a number of examples through the book of 'how not to do it', as well as how to do well. One station gives a dialogue illustrating bad history-taking technique in considerable detail (History 7: Headache). Here are ten other good ways of failing:

- Arrive for the exam late and looking untidy
- Forget to introduce yourself and don't ask the patient's name
- Be rude, brusque or inconsiderate towards the patient
- Suggest a diagnosis of cancer loudly and confidently in a patient's hearing
- Bombard the patient with closed questions and do not allow them to get in a word edgeways
- Examine a patient or perform a procedure without their consent
- Examine the patient in the wrong position and/or without undressing them appropriately
- Be careless with sharps and show a lack of awareness of infection risks
- Jump to a particular interpretation of some data and ignore all the examiner's attempts to steer you away from it
- Be 'cocky' with the examiner.

Doubtless some readers of this book will be resourceful enough to devise other failure strategies! Perhaps the commonest faults are to regard the examiner as 'out to fail you', and lose confidence because they question you aggressively. Most examiners are on your side. Sensible ones will try to coax every ounce of performance out of a weak student and test the limits of a strong one. Silly ones will do so in a bullying way.

How should I prepare for an OSCE?

Throughout your training, 'THINK SKILLS'.

- Make a list of the skills you need to acquire, and think which of them are relevant to the OSCE you are about to take.
- Read about them, and read around them. For example, revise the anatomy of the thyroid before going to the endocrine clinic to learn how to examine it. Read about the pathology of the thyroid so that you understand why it matters whether it is diffusely enlarged or nodular. That way, you will build up a solid understanding of what you are feeling and what you might feel on other occasions.
- Break a skill down to its component parts, write down a logical order in which to perform it, recite it to yourself as you practise the skill and repeat it in the bath until you have memorised it.
- Go over and over and over the skill 'in simulation' before you try your hand with patients. Skills laboratories are a valuable resource, but not the only one. Examining fellow students is a greatly underused way of learning. Have you ever considered that you can learn to recognise the A and V waves of the jugular venous pulse simply by asking your friend to lie on the floor and examining his neck?
- Try your hand at the skill on patients, and analyse what is difficult about it. Ask a doctor to help. You will make far better use of their scant time if you

say *'I'm having difficulty with the ankle jerk and I'm not sure if I've got the positioning right'* than if you say *'I'm hopeless at neurological examination; please give me a teaching session on it'*.

- Try to second-guess the exam. This is illustrated in the Examination stations (Chapter 4) where we have indicated what diseases are commonly available to examiners, and in what directions they may 'extend' you on particular skills.

OTHER TYPES OF EXAM

There is nothing magical about OSCEs. All types of clinical exam test the same skills and you can apply just the same principles in preparing for them. To make that point, we depart from classical OSCE format on a few occasions in this book (e.g. History 6: Erectile dysfunction). Where we describe histories from 'real' patients (e.g. History 8: Collapse: Communication 11: Respond to a patient's distress), the underlying skill could apply equally well to a traditional long or short case as to an OSCE or OSLER (see next paragraph) exam.

OSCEs may be 'flavour of the month', but they are not the last word in examinations. The strength of an OSCE is that it allows a wide range of knowledge and skills to be tested in an efficient and reliable way; however, you need to be able to unravel complex and unique circumstances as well as stereotyped ones to be competent in medicine. The OSLER (**O**bjective **S**tructured **L**ong **E**xamination **R**ecord, e.g. Examination 25: Examine the skin) is an example of an alternative assessment that uses OSCE principles in the complex setting of 'a real patient with real problems'. Don't be blinkered in your exam preparations. Understand the principles of good performance and apply them to whatever type of assessment you are facing.

THIS BOOK

Contents

This book is based on a careful analysis of the skills needed at graduation. It is not complete, and is biased towards medicine. As you go through other clerkships, be aware of the other skills that are required of you and build up your repertoire using the same principles.

Presentation

We have grouped the stations into six chapters by the type of skill. In each of those chapters, the skills are listed system-by-system. There is a tab at the edge of each page indicating the type of skill and the relevant system. That way you can either learn a particular type of skill across the systems, or go through the skills pertaining to an individual system. Table 1.2 lists the contents of the book by system and type of skill. The book is indexed so that you can look up a theme (e.g. consent) and pick out all the stations where that theme emerges. We have

Table 1.2 The contents of this book

Skill	Cardiovascular	Respiratory	Gastrointestinal	Genitourinary	Neurological	Haematological	Endocrine/ metabolic	Locomotor	Infectious diseases	General
History	• Chest pain • Present the history of chest pain	• Cough and breathlessness	• Diarrhoea	• Abdominal pain • Erectile dysfunction	• Headache • Collapse	• Skin rash	• Thirst and polyuria	• Back pain		• Pyrexia • Lethargy • Alcohol history
Examination	• Measure blood pressure • Heart examination • Peripheral vascular examination	• Respiratory examination 1 • Respiratory examination 2	• Examine the abdomen • Rectal examination	• Male genital examination	• Examine higher cortical function • Vision • Hearing • Examine the lower cranial nerves • Examine the sensory system in the arms • Sensory examination • Examine the motor system in the arms • Examine the motor system in the legs • Examine coordination	• Lymph node examination	• Examine the neck	• Examine the spine • Shoulder examination • Examine the hands • Examine the hip • Examine the knee		• Examine the skin
Interpretation	• Urea and electrolytes	• Chest radiograph		• Urinalysis	• Cerebrospinal fluid	• Blood count	• Deliberate self-harm • Weight gain and hypertension	• Acute arthropathy		

Table 1.2 (cont'd)

Skill	Cardiovascular	Respiratory	Gastrointestinal	Genitourinary	Neurological	Haematological	Endocrine/metabolic	Locomotor	Infectious diseases	General
Procedures	Record an ECG Intravenous injection Advanced life support	Diagnostic pleural aspiration Write a prescription	Nasogastric intubation	Urethral catheterisation Venous cannulation		Blood transfusion	Finger-prick blood glucose measurement	Aspirate knee joint		Basic life support Venepuncture Suture skin Arterial blood sampling Death certification
Communication	Explain statin therapy Discuss a 'do not resuscitate' order	Teach inhaler technique Discuss with a carer	Endoscopy	Explain 24 h urine collection	Lumbar puncture	Break bad news	Respond to a patient's dissatisfaction Cross-cultural communication	Respond to a patient's distress	Discuss HIV testing	Give information to a patient
Attitudes		Criminal activity			A problem with epilepsy	A difficult haematemesis			Risk of infection	Giving information by telephone Problems with your colleague A cry for help? Terminal care

11

offered a number of possible 'do it yourself' OSCE circuits in Chapter 2 so that you (with or without your friends) can construct specimen OSCEs according to the particular exam you are facing, and use the text to revise and judge your performance.

Layout of individual stations

At the head of each station, we have used a star rating to indicate its complexity:

– Basic   *
– Intermediate   **
– Advanced   ***

These equate roughly with your clinical year; stations with higher star markings are likely to test you on abnormal pathology/'real' patients. Where a basic physical examination skill could be 'extended' to abnormal physical signs, the star rating will show a range.

We have indicated the type of examination we had in mind for each station, but you should not take that too literally. It is the description of the skill that you should concentrate on. Finally, we have included suggestions for further practice.

How to use it

Students who fail OSCEs are rarely plain clumsy. They have usually:

● Underestimated the importance of learning skills and concentrated too much on cramming facts.
● Failed to draw their skills and knowledge together in the way illustrated throughout this book.

It follows that, to excel in the OSCE, you should learn skills and knowledge in tandem. In practical terms, start your OSCE revision on day 1 of the clinical course and, whenever you are book-learning, think of the **practical** application of what you are learning about. Use the OSCE as an incentive and it will become a pathway to the competence to which you must surely aspire.

Core skill/principle boxes

We have summarised the content of the book in these boxes. If you refer to them regularly, the book will serve as a textbook of clinical skills as well as an exam revision guide. The boxes are listed in Table 1.3.

Table 1.3 Core skill boxes

Skill type	Title	Page no.
History	• Communicating with a patient in order to take a history	28
	• Structuring a history in an OSCE exam	29
	• Applying knowledge while taking a history	29
	• Presenting a history	32
	• Asking personal details	42
	• Responding to a patient's talkativeness	54
	• Taking an alcohol history	71
Examination	• Measurement of blood pressure	79
	• Examination of the heart	81
	• Examination of the peripheral vascular system	87
	• Examination of the respiratory system	89
	• Detection and interpretation of respiratory signs	92
	• Abdominal examination	96
	• Rectal examination	101
	• Examination of the male genitalia	103
	• Examination of higher cognitive function	105
	• Visual examination	109
	• Examination of hearing	112
	• Lower cranial nerve examination	114
	• Sensory examination of the arms	117
	• Sensory examination of the legs	122
	• Examining real patients	123
	• Motor examination of arms	125
	• Motor examination of the legs	129
	• Coordination	133
	• Lymph node examination	136
	• Examination of thyroid gland	139
	• Examination of the spine	142
	• Examination of the shoulder	144
	• Joint examination of hands	147
	• Hip examination	150
	• Knee examination	153
	• Skin examination	157
Data interpretation	• Interpretation of urea and electrolytes	162
	• Interpretation of a chest radiograph	165
	• Interpretation of urine tests	169
	• Interpretation of CSF results	172
	• Interpretation of full blood count	175
	• Assessment of deliberate self-harm	177
Procedures	• Recording an ECG	190
	• Reading an ECG	192
	• Intravenous drug injection	194
	• Diagnostic pleural aspiration	201
	• Interpretation of pleural fluid	202
	• Completing a prescription chart	206
	• Pass a nasogastric tube	207
	• Urethral catheterisation	209
	• Venous cannulation	212
	• Choosing an intravenous fluid	214

Table 1.3 *(cont'd)*

Skill type	Title	Page no.
	● Blood transfusion	218
	● Finger-prick blood glucose measurement	221
	● Knee joint aspiration	222
	● Interpretation of joint aspirate	223
	● Venepuncture	227
	● Skin suturing	229
	● Radial arterial puncture	231
	● Interpreting blood gas measurements	233
	● Completing a death certificate	237
	● Choosing which patients to refer to the coroner	237
Communication	● Reaching agreement about treatment	246
	● Discussing resuscitation status with a patient	251
	● Teaching a patient a procedure	253
	● Discussion with a carer	255
	● Responding to resistant behaviour	260
	● How to give an effective explanation	263
	● Obtaining informed consent	266
	● Breaking bad news	270
	● Responding to anger	275
	● Communicating through an interpreter	278
	● Cross-cultural communication	280
	● Responding to emotionally charged situations	282
	● Discussion in preparation for an HIV test	284
Attitudes	● Dealing with potentially criminal incidents	295
	● Epilepsy and the law	297
	● Respect for autonomy	299
	● Handling information concerning risk to others	302
	● Health of your colleagues	307
	● Competency	309
	● Managing dying patients	312

CHAPTER 2

Specimen OSCEs

Introduction

There are 84 stations in this book, ranging from simple skills that can be tested in a preclinical anatomy or physiology department to complex skills involving patients with disease. To introduce some challenge to your revision, we have arranged them into a number of examinations of increasing complexity. We have assumed a 5-year medical course with:

- Limited clinical exposure and skills teaching in the first 2 years.
- A concentration on basic clinical skills and cardiorespiratory and gastrointestinal disease in Year 3 (corresponding to junior medicine and surgery).
- More detailed and specialised learning in Year 4, including locomotor and neurological disease.
- Preparation for practice and acquisition of complex clinical management skills in Year 5.

Each specimen examination tests a variety of types of skill, and the different body systems, to mimic the variety that you will meet in real exams. If you would prefer to concentrate your revision on a particular skill type or a particular system, skip directly to Chapters 3–8, which are organised along those lines.

SKILLS EXAMS EARLY IN THE COURSE (YEARS 1–2)

Medical schools differ greatly in the amount of skills teaching they offer in the early years. If you have not been taught skills, you are most unlikely to be tested on them. Exams A and B include skills that **could** be tested at this stage of training.

Exam A			
Skill	System	Type	Comment
Explain 24-h urine Page 262	Genitourinary	Communication	Communication skills could be tested on a procedure like this that requires little specialised knowledge
Chest radiograph Page 164	Respiratory	Data	At this stage, the emphasis would be on recognising anatomical landmarks rather than disease
Measure blood pressure Page 79	Cardiovascular	Examination	
Venepuncture Page 227	General	Procedure	

SPECIMEN OSCEs

Exam A *(cont'd)*

Skill	System	Type	Comment
Lower cranial nerves Page 114	Neurological	Examination	Examination of individual nerves could be taught and tested as an exercise in applied anatomy

Exam B

Skill	System	Type	Comment
Teach inhaler technique Page 252	Respiratory	Communication	
Measure blood glucose Page 220	Endocrine/ Metabolic	Procedure/data	This could be used both to test skill at a procedure and knowledge of basic biochemistry
Vision Page 109	Neurological	Examination	Another test of applied anatomy/physiology
Record an ECG Page 190	Cardiovascular	Procedure	
Basic life support Page 224	General	Procedure	A skill that many lay people acquire and one that will certainly be expected of a junior medical student

SKILLS EXAM IN YEAR 3 (JUNIOR MEDICINE/SURGERY)

See Chapter 1, Table 1.1 (page 4) for a detailed specimen examination. There is likely to be a strong emphasis on basic history-taking at this stage in your training. Physical examination will probably be tested on volunteers, to demonstrate basic clinical method rather than skill at eliciting abnormal physical signs. Here are two more short 'circuses':

Exam C

Skill	System	Type
Examine the abdomen Page 96	Gastrointestinal	Examination
Cough and breathlessness Page 33	Respiratory	History

Exam C *(cont'd)*

Skill	System	Type
Present the history Page 31	Respiratory	History
Cerebrospinal fluid Page 171	Neurological	Data
Male genital examination Page 103	Genitourinary	Examination

Exam D

Skill	System	Type
Heart examination Page 81	Cardiovascular	Examination
Lethargy Page 67	General	History
Present the history Page 31	General	History
Urinalysis Page 168	Genitourinary	Data
Examine the spine Page 142	Locomotor	Examination

SKILLS EXAM IN THE MIDDLE CLINICAL YEAR

By this stage, you should be consolidating and broadening your skills and beginning to diagnose 'the abnormal'. You will have studied some more specialised clinical disciplines such as rheumatology, ophthalmology and neurology.

Exam E

Skill	System	Type
Alcohol history Page 71	General	History
Present the history Page 31	General	History
Lymph node examination Page 136	Haematological	Examination

Exam E *(cont'd)*

Skill	System	Type
Intravenous injection Page 193	Procedure	Cardiovascular
Blood count Page 174	Haematological	Data
Hearing Page 112	Neurological	Examination
Thirst and polyuria Page 59	Endocrine/Metabolic	History
Examine the hands Page 147	Locomotor	Examination
Aspirate knee joint Page 222	Locomotor	Procedure

Exam F

Skill	System	Type
Headache Page 44	Neurological	History
Present the history Page 31	Neurological	History
Heart examination Page 81	Cardiovascular	Examination
Suture skin Page 229	Procedure	General
Deliberate self-harm Page 177	Endocrine/Metabolic	Data
Examine the motor system in the arms Page 123	Neurological	Examination
Skin rash Page 56	Haematological	History
Shoulder examination Page 144	Locomotor	Examination
Venous cannulation Page 212	Genitourinary	Procedure

FINAL SKILLS EXAMINATION

You are likely to be tested on physical examination of patients with abnormal signs, more complex communication and attitudinal issues, procedures that you will be called upon to perform as a house officer and histories. Some stations are likely to test skills that you were taught in the earlier years of training.

Exam G		
Skill	System	Type
Examine the skin Page 156	General	Examination
Explain statin therapy Page 243	Cardiovascular	Communication
Blood transfusion Page 215	Haematological	Procedure
Criminal activity Page 294	Respiratory	Attitude
Sensory examination Page 121	Neurological	Examination
Death certification Page 235	General	Procedure
Back pain Page 62	Endocrine/Metabolic	History
Present the history Page 31	Locomotor	History

Exam H		
Skill	System	Type
Examine the hip Page 150	Locomotor	Examination
Endoscopy Page 258	Gastrointestinal	Communication
Write a prescription Page 204	Respiratory	Procedure
Risk of infection Page 301	Infectious diseases	Attitude
Peripheral vascular examination Page 86	Cardiovascular	Examination

Exam H *(cont'd)*

Skill	System	Type
Arterial blood sampling Page 231	General	Procedure
Abdominal pain Page 38	Genitourinary	History
Present the history Page 31	Locomotor	History

Exam I

Skill	System	Type
Examine higher cortical function Page 105	Neurological	Examination
Discuss HIV testing Page 284	Infectious diseases	Communication
Advanced life support Page 197	Cardiovascular	Procedure
Problems with your colleague Page 306	General	Attitude
Examine the neck Page 139	Endocrine/Metabolic	Examination
Diagnostic pleural aspiration Page 200	Respiratory	Procedure
Diarrhoea Page 35	Gastrointestinal	History
Present the history Page 31	Gastrointestinal	History

STRUCTURED ORAL EXAMINATION

What some medical schools call an OSCE, others call a viva or structured oral. This tests your ability to apply knowledge, and may also test your attitudes. If you are coming up to a viva, you could use the following stations to support your revision:

History

Data interpretation

All the stations are in structured oral format.

Procedures

Communication

Attitudes

All the stations are in structured oral format.

LONG AND SHORT CASE FORMAT

Although this book is orientated towards the OSCE style of examination, it can help you prepare for more traditional examinations, both by giving a description of core clinical skills and describing techniques and approaches that are very relevant to long and short cases. For example:

History

Examination

All stations describe the core clinical skills that you will be called upon to demonstrate in traditional clinical examinations; many of them are extended into the common pathologies that you will encounter in such examinations.

CHAPTER 3

History skills

Introduction

History-taking is central to medicine and will figure prominently in OSCEs. More than in any other type of station, there is a limited set of core skills that must be tailored to a wide range of situations. This section starts with a brief general introduction first to **taking** and then to **presenting** a history and then gives an example of each (History 1: Chest pain, and History 2: Present chest pain history). The main skills are described in four core skill boxes in those two stations; the stations that follow, describe how you could apply those skills to a range of clinical problems. Most stations involve interviewing standardised patients (see Introductory chapter, page 3 for an explanation).

THE SKILL OF HISTORY-TAKING

There are three components:

- The PROCESS of good communication
- The STRUCTURE of the medical interview
- The KNOWLEDGE CONTENT relevant to the symptom or situation.

Communication process

The dialogue in History 1: Chest pain, has been written out in detail to illustrate a number of points of good practice; in contrast, History 7: Headache, illustrates one way of not doing it. In the second example, the student is concerned to use the short time of the OSCE to extract 'the facts' at all costs. She does so at the expense of demonstrating her skill as a communicator, and shows no concern for the patient. The examiner may be as concerned about the quality of communication as the factual content of the interview – and patients will certainly be. Where dialogues have been written out in full (History 1, 6 & 8), you should not attempt to repeat them verbatim. No two people communicate in the same way and you will come across as a complete sham if you adopt large chunks of another person's language; observe other peoples' style and then see what works well for you. The core skill of communicating well during history-taking is tabulated in a core skill box, page 28.

Interview structure

History 1, page 26, shows how a student can use limited time well by following a clearly defined structure and focussing on relevant information; the core skill is shown in a box on page 28. Not all interviews are straightforward. Patients often tell you things in what feels a chaotic order, dodging from one 'compartment' of the history to another. You should certainly not use any structure as a 'straight-jacket' but you can use your communication skills to order the interview:

- *I was very interested in what you were saying a moment ago about your brother's heart attack, may I ask you a little more about that? How old was he when it happened?*

- *May I take just a moment to summarise what you've told me so I can check that I've understood everything that is important to you?*

Remember that no-one can expect you to take a comprehensive history in 5 minutes.

Knowledge content

You need knowledge as well as skill to do well in OSCEs. The trick is to apply your knowledge so that you take a focussed (or 'problem-orientated') history. A problem-orientated approach to the knowledge content of a short history is summarised in a core skill box on page 29.

The pages that follow run through a variety of history taking stations, building on the points about communication and structure discussed above and helping you think about the knowledge specific to each station and the direction in which the examiner's questions may take you.

To prepare for an OSCE, think out which histories are most likely to appear in the exam and practise them first in role-play with a friend (that way, both of you benefit) and then with patients on the wards. Ask a fellow student to observe you and criticise your performance. There is no substitute for clinical experience to build your confidence and competence.

THE SKILL OF PRESENTING A HISTORY

The dialogue in History 2: Present the history of chest pain, illustrates the characteristics of a good presentation. The box on page 32 describes the core skill. Here are some general points:

- Listen very carefully to what the examiner asks. In the example on page 31, the examiner made it easy. Sometimes, they may throw you by saying *'tell me the diagnosis'*, or worse. In all events, DO WHAT YOU'RE TOLD, but see if you can exceed the examiner's expectations.
- Try to cover as much ground as possible without the examiner having to speak. By the time he did so in the specimen dialogue, he would have been deciding on honours points, not pass or failure.

THE USE OF NOTES

You will probably want to make notes as you take your histories. You would be well advised to make them in the order you expect to give your presentation rather than the order the patient gives you the information. The principles of good doctor–patient communication dictate that information will come out in the patient's order, not yours. However, the fact that the social history comes out before the history of the presenting complaint does not oblige you to write them down in that order. Use a large piece of paper to give you plenty of space to structure the key points into the order in which you plan to present them. If your notes are chaotic, your presentation will be chaotic as well.

HISTORY 1	**Chest pain**	
Level:	*	
Setting:	Middle-aged female standardised patient seated in a room with a desk	
Time:	5 min	

TASK

E – *Please take a history from this patient. You will be asked to present your history at the next station.*

RESPONSE

S – *(Makes eye contact and shakes patient's hand.)*
– *Good morning, my name is Briony. I am a third year medical student. Can you tell me your name?*

P – Joan Smith.

S – *(Sits across corner of desk from patient and smiles.)*
– *May I take a history from you?*

P – Yes.

S – *May I ask your age and occupation?*

P – I'm 55. I've finished work.

S – *What seems to be the problem?*

P – I keep getting this pain in my chest.

S – *Pain in your chest?*

P – Yes, it began when I was on holiday last September. It was quite a climb up from the beach to the hotel and I felt as though there was a heavy weight on my chest.

S – *Can you tell me a little more about that incident?*

P – I was carrying a heavy picnic bag. I put it down and sat at the side of the road for 5 minutes and the pain eased off. I felt quite short of breath but it soon passed.

S – *Can you describe the pain in more detail?*

P – As I said, it was a heavy weight. It was across the front of my chest. I felt a tightness in my throat and a sort of heaviness in my left arm, and I felt short of breath. It all settled in just a few minutes, and I took it slowly the rest of the way to the hotel.

S – *And what has been happening since then?*

P – I didn't think any more of it until I was doing the shopping a couple of months ago, rushing to get home for lunch when the same happened again. Since then, I've had the chest tightness when I hurry or walk up hills. It seems to be coming more often. I'm beginning to wonder – there was a woman at work who got angina and she dropped dead with a heart attack.

S – *So you're worried about what this pain means to your health.*

P – Yes.

S – *That's very understandable after the experience with the person you know at work. Can I check that I have got all the details straight? Since your holiday last year, you've had a heavy pressure across the front of your chest, a tightness in your throat, a heaviness in your left arm and breathlessness when your hurry or walk uphill. It seems to be coming on more readily and you're worried about the possibility of heart disease.*

P – Yes, it's been really bothering me for the last 2 months; and sometimes I get the breathlessness without the pain when I hurry.

S – *Thank you for that extra information. Have you noticed if the pain is affected by the weather; what about cold days or strong winds?*

P – Yes, it's definitely worse on cold days.

S – *May I ask some more general questions about your health?*

P – Yes.

S – *Have you had any other illnesses?*

P – Only childhood ones. I hadn't seen the doctor since my second daughter was born.

S – *Have you ever been told you had high blood pressure or a high level of cholesterol in your blood?*

P – No.

S – *Are you on any tablets for this chest pain or anything else; hormone replacement treatment for example?*

S – No.

S – *Is there any heart disease in your family; for example, have your parents, brothers, sisters or children had heart disease?*

P – My mother died of a heart attack.

S – *How old was she?*

P – 68.

S – *Do you smoke.*

P – Not now.

S – *When did you stop, and how much did you smoke?*

P – 20 cigarettes a day, until that women at work dropped dead. That was 5 years ago.

S – *It sounds as though that incident alarmed you.*

P – You're telling me it did.

S – *How much alcohol do you drink?*

P – I don't drink at all.

S – *When did you finish work and what did you do?*

P – January this year. Just cleaning work.

S – *Was that as a result of this problem?*

P   No, I was offered early retirement.

E – *You have just one minute left.*

S – *Do you get any pains in your calves, for example when you walk?*

P – No.

S – *Thank you for giving me such a clear description of this pain which is causing you so much concern. You've also told me that that you used to smoke, that you*

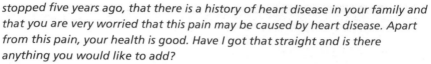

stopped five years ago, that there is a history of heart disease in your family and that you are very worried that this pain may be caused by heart disease. Apart from this pain, your health is good. Have I got that straight and is there anything you would like to add?

P – No.

S – *I would really need to examine you before reaching a diagnosis but are there any questions you would like to ask me?*

P – No.

S – *Thank you again, and I hope the doctor is able to sort out that pain for you. Goodbye. (Shakes hands again.)*

This dialogue is complementary to the 'Introduction to history taking'; read the core skill boxes carefully and use this dialogue as a model of how you might tackle other history-taking stations.

This station tests knowledge of chest pain and angina. A good student will not be content with diagnosing angina but will see it as a manifestation of vascular disease. Chest pain is one of the commonest causes of hospital admission so you

---

Core skill: Communicating with a patient in order to take a history

1. The setting:
   - You and the patient should be comfortably seated at the same level in a way that allows you to face and observe one another without the desk as a barrier between you.

2. Non-verbal communication:
   - No matter how tense you feel, try to retain a friendly, attentive manner. Use a smile and a handshake to establish the relationship; be aware of your posture and gestures during the consultation.

3. Introduce yourself, establish the patient's identity and ask permission to take the history.

4. Questioning:
   - Like the student in History station 1, make good use of open questions (*can you describe the pain in more detail?*). To obtain a clear and precise history, use closed questions to clarify what the patient has said, or to obtain pieces of factual information that the patient did not volunteer. Save closed questions until the patient has had a chance to tell their tale.

5. Identify and respond to the patient's perceptions and concerns (see Communication 11: Respond to a patient's distress).

6. Summarise periodically and at the end of the interview.

7. Give the patient a chance to add information or ask questions.

8. Finish by thanking the patient.

Core skill: Structuring a history in an OSCE exam

1. Introductions and consent.

2. Identify the main symptoms/problems.

3. Use about half your time to obtain a detailed history of those symptoms.

4. Use your interpretation of the problem (see Core skill box: Applying knowledge) to take a **relevant** previous medical history, family history, drug and alcohol history, social history and systems review.

5. Allow yourself time to think before presenting to the examiner.

6. Remember always to 'wind up' with the patient, even if the bell goes!

---

would be foolish to attend a clinical OSCE without the basic knowledge that underpins an appropriate history. In this case, the description was so typical of angina that, when time became short, Briony asked questions about vascular

---

Core skill: Applying knowledge while taking a history

1. Identify the main symptom(s).

2. Obtain information relevant to that symptom; in the case of a pain, clarify its nature, site, radiation, and precipitating and alleviating factors. There is an analogous set of information for other common symptoms such as collapse (History 8) and diarrhoea (History 4)

3. Think of the different causes of that particular symptom. In the case of chest pain, think of the structures within the chest that can give rise to pain (heart, oesophagus, pericardium, pleura, intercostal nerves, muscles and bones) and seek symptoms referrable to them.

4. If a diagnosis seems likely, think of the risk factors predisposing to that disease; in the case of ischaemic chest pain, ask about family history, smoking and hyperlipidaemia.

5. Think also of diseases that may complicate or be associated with the main problem; for example, ask about stroke and peripheral vascular disease in a patient with ischaemic heart disease.

6. Think of possible effects of the disease on the patient, particularly occupational issues. Ischaemic chest pain matters more to a long distance truck driver than a non-driver.

7. Only ask about completely unrelated symptoms or problems if you have time on your hands.

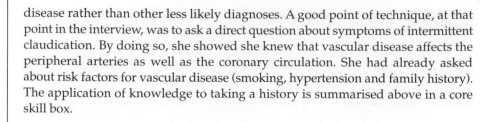

disease rather than other less likely diagnoses. A good point of technique, at that point in the interview, was to ask a direct question about symptoms of intermittent claudication. By doing so, she showed she knew that vascular disease affects the peripheral arteries as well as the coronary circulation. She had already asked about risk factors for vascular disease (smoking, hypertension and family history). The application of knowledge to taking a history is summarised above in a core skill box.

SUGGESTIONS FOR FURTHER PRACTICE

You must be very experienced in taking histories from patients with chest pain.

Ask a colleague to observe how well you communicate with patients while taking histories

- See how far you can go without asking a single closed question.
- How good are you at listening attentively and allowing the patient to speak?
- Do you know how to respond with empathy if a patient expresses a negative emotion (see Communication 11)?

How good are you at structuring histories? Are you able to cope with patients who describe their symptoms in a chaotic order? Choose the vaguest and most talkative patient on your ward and ask a colleague to observe how you conduct the interview. Do a debrief together afterwards and develop strategies for structuring your interviews while remaining 'patient-centred'.

HISTORY 2	**Present the history of chest pain**
Level:	*
Setting:	You are asked to present the history to a seated examiner
Time:	5 min

TASK

E – *Please present the history of the patient you have just seen.*

RESPONSE

S – *Mrs Joan Smith is a 55-year-old retired cleaner who complains of a pressing chest pain radiating to the throat and associated with heaviness in the left arm. Her first episode was 6 months ago and it has been coming with increasing frequency for the last 2 months. It is brought on by exertion, particularly carrying shopping bags and walking uphill, and is relieved after about 2 minutes of rest. It is worse in cold weather. She is breathless with the pain and has some exertional dyspnoea. As far as risk factors for ischaemic heart disease are concerned, she has no history of hypertension or hyperlipidaemia but has a family history of ischaemic heart disease – her mother died at 68 of a heart attack – and she smoked 20 cigarettes a day until 5 years ago. Her health is otherwise good. She has no other past history, no stroke or TIAs and no symptoms of intermittent claudication. I think she has a typical history of angina. That is what she thinks is wrong with her and she is worried that she may drop dead with a heart attack. Having examined her for other signs of arterial disease or underlying heart disease, I would request an ECG and measure her fasting lipids and glucose. Unless the ECG gave a clear diagnosis, I would request an Exercise Test.*

E – *I was interested to hear you say that you would examine her for signs of underlying heart disease, what diseases other than ischaemic heart disease might you find on examination of a patient with angina?*

S – *I would want to check her pulse rate – a tachycardia such as atrial fibrillation could cause angina by increasing cardiac work. I would look for signs of aortic stenosis, including a slow rising, low-volume pulse, a narrow pulse pressure, a thrusting apex beat and a mid-systolic murmur in the aortic area radiating into the carotid arteries.*

The introduction to this section (page 25) and the core skill box below describe the features of a good presentation, using this dialogue as an example. Note how Briony has given a clear and concise presentation, for which she is guaranteed good marks. She has taken the initiative to present her knowledge about cardiovascular disease, again without waiting for too much prompting from the examiner.

> ## Core skill: Presenting a history
>
> 1. Structure it clearly.
>
> 2. Express it economically:
>   - In station 2, the largely negative previous history is put across in just a few words, concentrating on **relevant** negatives. That allows time for the examiner to ask extra questions at the end and increase the score.
>
> 3. Show signs of thought:
>   - Early in the presentation in station 2, the student shows that she recognises the diagnosis and implies that the presence of risk factors is important both in weighting the likelihood of the diagnosis and in determining management.
>
> 4. Report the patient's perceptions and concerns:
>   - In the specimen dialogue, the student identifies information that would be useful in managing the patient and, in doing so, shows concern for her.
>
> 5. Offer a diagnosis and suggest what to look for in the examination:
>   - Many diagnoses can be made from the history and frequently the examination will be negative (likely in this case) but you can show your 'problem orientation' by stating what examination findings would confirm your working diagnosis.
>
> 6. Offer an investigation and/or management plan.

As you get towards the end of a history presentation, the examiner could ask you anything relevant to the station. You will gain extra marks if you demonstrate factual knowledge but should not lose any if you are stumped by the questions. It is inadvisable to spin out your presentation to stop the examiner having time to question you because a slow and wordy presentation will not attract good marks.

SUGGESTIONS FOR FURTHER PRACTICE

- Practise writing concise, structured notes on your histories with the key points in a sensible order for presentation.
- Practise turning the histories you take into concise presentations. To start with, allow yourself more than 5 minutes, and work with another student. With experience, do it in a shorter time and ask a house officer to act as your examiner. Best of all, present cases on consultant ward rounds; by comparison, an OSCE may seem informal and non-threatening.
- Try to develop confidence in making diagnoses. This will increase the quality of your presentations and show your examiners (and bosses) that you are more than a passive recipient and regurgitator of facts.

HISTORY 3	**Cough and breathlessness**
Level:	*
Setting:	A standardised patient
Time:	10 min

TASK

You are asked to take and then present a history from a 44-year-old woman who reports cough and dyspnoea. At the end of your presentation, the examiner asks you what physical signs would distinguish between the possible causes.

RESPONSE

Your history should tease out the possible causes of these two symptoms. The core skill box on page 29 discusses how you can apply knowledge while taking a history. Table 3.1 shows a differential diagnosis in this case, together with other relevant symptoms and signs.

E – *Suppose the patient had cough but no dyspnoea; what other causes might you consider?*

Causes to consider include:

- Smoker's cough
- ACE-inhibitor treatment
- Inhaled foreign body
- Post-nasal drip
- Gastro-oesophageal reflux
- Habit/psychogenic cough.

Having been asked that question, don't wait to be asked for a differential diagnosis, key physical signs and appropriate investigations. Phrase your reply to the examiner: *Diagnoses which should be considered include … When examining the patient, I would look for …. I would arrange a …*

SUGGESTIONS FOR FURTHER PRACTICE

Get plenty of practice at taking histories from patients with common medical problems like cough and dyspnoea but don't be satisfied just with recording the details. Examine the patients, look at their chest X-rays yourself and find the results of other investigations. Make up your own mind about the diagnosis. That way, you will come to exams confident in your diagnostic skills.

Table 3.1 Causes of cough and dyspnoea

	Asthma/COPD	Bronchiectasis	Ca bronchus	Acute lower respiratory tract infection	Heart failure
Length of history	Variable	Likely to be longstanding	May be recent and progressively worsening	Likely to be very recent history	Variable
Sputum	Variable; may be none, may be yellow/green	Large volume; may be purulent. Haemoptysis may occur	Variable; haemoptysis may occur	None or purulent; haemoptysis may occur	Typically frothy and may be blood-stained; may be no sputum
Associated symptom(s)[1]	Wheeze		Weight loss	Symptoms of fever	Ankle swelling
Other points to ask about in history[2]	Allergies Family history	Previous respiratory illness; e.g. childhood whooping cough			May give history of ischaemic heart disease, hypertension or valvular disease
Key physical sign(s)	Wheeze	Localised crackles Finger clubbing may occur	No single key sign; finger clubbing may occur	Signs of consolidation: bronchial breathing, increased vocal resonance and tactile vocal fremitus, dullness to percussion	Enlarged heart, raised jugular venous pressure, oedema, tachycardia, basal crackles
Key investigation	Peak flow; reduced	Chest X-ray; may show abnormal lung markings	Chest X-ray; may show tumour mass or other changes	Chest X-ray; likely to show infiltrates	Chest X-ray: cardiomegaly and upper lobe venous diversion. May also show pleural effusions and fluid in the fissures

[1]Orthopnoea is classically associated with heart failure, but any cause of breathlessness may worsen on lying flat.
[2]Smoking is a risk factor for all of these diseases. You must take a smoking history, but you cannot distinguish between them on the strength of the smoking history.

HISTORY 4	**Diarrhoea**
Level:	*
Setting:	Take a history from a standardised patient
Time:	5 min

TASK

It turns out that the patient's presenting complaint is diarrhoea and you have to explore it as thoroughly as possible in 5 minutes.

RESPONSE

This is another opportunity to put into practice the principles discussed in the introduction to history-taking skills. To be specific, you must work within the **structure** of the medical history, use good **communication skills** to 'hear the patient's story', and **apply knowledge** to focus and enquire about key factual details. It illustrates how a knowledgeable student could compress the lengthy process of 'taking a complete history' into very limited time.

Your history should include:

1. A detailed description of the diarrhoea itself.
2. A chronological description of its onset and events related to it.
3. Enquiry into background factors that might explain the cause of the diarrhoea or have resulted from it.
4. An enquiry into related symptoms.

Diarrhoea

A good starter is to ask the patient what he means by diarrhoea or to describe his diarrhoea. Pay attention to:

- Frequency of bowel action
- Timing through the day and night
- Constancy or variability of the diarrhoea
- Description of the motion
    Volume
    Appearance
- Presence of:
    Blood
    Slime
    Symptoms of steatorrhoea; typically a pale, greasy motion which may stain the toilet bowl, floats and requires the toilet to be flushed several times
- Faecal incontinence
- Relationship of bowel actions to eating

- Feelings of:
    Incomplete evacuation
    'Tenesmus'; feeling a need to evacuate when the rectum is empty
- Pain; if present, get a detailed description of the pain and how its time-course relates to the diarrhoea.

Chronological description of the diarrhoea and events related to it

Students tend to rush on to this phase of the history without obtaining a clear description of the symptom itself. That applies to many aspects of history-taking; see History 7: Headache, for another example. Often, the chronology and the description of the presenting symptom are inextricably linked but be sure that you clarify **both**. A good starter for this phase would be: *Can you take me back to when you first experienced diarrhoea?* Obtain a clear description of:

- The time-course of the illness
- Any obvious precipitant
- Factors which exacerbate or relieve the diarrhoea
- Any symptoms affecting other parts of the gastrointestinal tract (e.g. nausea, vomiting).

Also, get a feeling for whether the patient is 'ill' and listen carefully for any associated symptoms such as:

- Weight loss
- Fever
- Symptoms affecting other systems.

Background factors

Previous medical history

- Any relevant illnesses, including operations, and hospital admissions.

Family history

- Any relevant gastrointestinal disease.

Social history

- Disease in other family members or co-habitants; that is particularly relevant if the history suggests infective diarrhoea. You may need to go into a lot of detail about who in the household ate what and when. You may also need to enquire in depth about sources of food and how it was stored.
- Living conditions.
- Foreign travel.
- Other aspects of social history may also be relevant; if, for example, the patient were a man without a regular heterosexual partner who had diarrhoea, was ill and losing weight, enquiry into his sexual orientation and habits would be relevant (on suspicion of AIDS). See History 6: Erectile dysfunction.

Drug and alcohol history

Enquire about:

- Antibiotic therapy (antibiotic-induced diarrhoea)
- Purgatives (purgative abuse)
- Any other use of prescription or non-prescription drugs.

Enquiry into related symptoms

Diseases associated with diarrhoea can cause symptoms in any system. The 'problem-orientated clinician' will have asked key questions when exploring the presenting complaint. As a general rule, you should end your histories with a careful systems review to 'screen' for symptoms not detected by the history. If you have one or more diagnoses in mind, you should also use the systems review to seek out any symptoms that might support those diagnoses or make them unlikely.

SUGGESTIONS FOR FURTHER PRACTICE

Prepare a table with 10 (or however many you have the energy for) important causes of diarrhoea and tabulate features in the various sections of the history which would help in making the diagnosis.

HISTORY SKILLS

HISTORY 5	**Abdominal pain**
Level:	*
Setting:	You have misjudged your timing and only have 3 minutes to go. You have established that the 68-year-old patient has right loin pain that has been present for some weeks. The examiner, seeing that you have nowhere near enough information to suggest a diagnosis (which is needed for the next station) intervenes to help you out
Time:	10 min

TASK

E – *Time is short. I would like you to suggest five causes for this patient's pain. For each cause, suggest one specific symptom or sign that, if present, would strongly support that diagnosis.*

RESPONSE

An experienced diagnostician will know which symptoms are particularly helpful in making which diagnoses. A 'specific' symptom/sign is one that may not be present in every patient with a particular disease but, if present, makes the diagnosis very likely. Vague symptoms such as tiredness are almost never as valuable as that. Think carefully which symptom you volunteer.

When asked to give causes for a pain in a particular location, think of the

Table 3.2 Symptoms that differentiate different causes of right loin pain

	Gallstones/ biliary colic	Renal stone	Colonic disease; e.g. tumour	Shingles	Nerve root entrapment
Nature of pain	Intermittent	Intermittent or constant	Intermittent or constant	Constant, burning	May be intermittent or constant
Associated clinical feature	May be precipitated by eating fatty food May radiate to the back	Haematuria	Change in bowel habit	Vesicular skin rash in dermatomal distribution	Pain worsened by movement
Investigation	Abdominal ultrasound	Abdominal ultrasound	Colonoscopy Barium enema Abdominal CT	None	Abnormal bony architecture on plain radiology

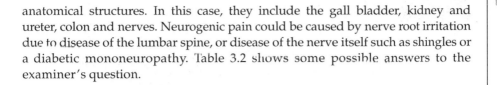

anatomical structures. In this case, they include the gall bladder, kidney and ureter, colon and nerves. Neurogenic pain could be caused by nerve root irritation due to disease of the lumbar spine, or disease of the nerve itself such as shingles or a diabetic mononeuropathy. Table 3.2 shows some possible answers to the examiner's question.

SUGGESTIONS FOR FURTHER PRACTICE

You should be absolutely confident with such a common symptom as abdominal pain. List as many causes as you can think of and the features that help distinguish between them. Draw up a list of other common symptoms and their cardinal clinical features. Seek out patients on your ward with abdominal pain and try to work out a differential diagnosis on clinical grounds.

HISTORY SKILLS

HISTORY 6 — Erectile dysfunction

Level:	***
Setting:	A medical long case. Mary is taking a history from Mr Hughes, a diabetic man of 55. After 15 minutes, she has obtained a full history of his diabetes and is confident that there will be ample time to examine him. She is aware that erectile dysfunction is a common problem among diabetic men
Time:	60 min

TASK

She sets herself the task of obtaining details of his sexual function.

RESPONSE

S – *Thank you for giving me such a complete description of your diabetes. I've asked you a lot of questions; are there any other things you would like to ask or tell me?*

Silence.

S – *We have plenty of time so please feel free to tell me anything about your health which concerns you.*

People with personal problems are most likely to volunteer them if they are given plenty of 'space'. This open questioning strategy has not elicited a sexual problem but has created a climate conducive to discussing personal problems.

S – *It is not uncommon for diabetic men to have difficulty in their sexual relations. Do you have any difficulty?*

Before asking a personal question, Mary has explained the reason for it. She has also indicated that it would be OK to admit to a sexual problem. Her question is delicately phrased, but direct.

P – Well, as a matter of fact, things aren't so good between the wife and myself.
S – *Not so good? Could you tell me more about that?*
P – It's embarrassing talking about it.
S – *I can understand that you find it embarrassing talking about something so personal; perhaps the fact that I am a woman makes it more difficult for you. I find it a little awkward asking you these questions myself, but it seems there is something worth talking about. Would you be willing to tell me more about it?*

She has acknowledged his embarrassment and made it easier for him by showing that she, also, finds the topic awkward.

P – It's the first time I've talked to anyone about it. The doctor didn't seem to have time to listen.

S – *Thank you for confiding in me. Could you tell me what the problem is?*

P – Don't seem to be able to keep it up like I used to.

S – *You have a problem maintaining an erection?*

P – Yes.

S – *Could you describe what happened when you last had intercourse?*

This factual question opens the way to a more precise description of the problem and is likely to elicit details about the quality of his erection, difficulty sustaining it, premature ejaculation or other sexual dysfunction. Mary should ask whether the problem is restricted to intercourse or whether morning erections are affected as well (suggesting organic erectile failure rather than dysfunction in their relationship).

S – *Have you maintained your interest in sex?*

This directs the discussion towards libido, and could lead into a discussion of psychological issues.

S – *Have you had other sexual partners?*

P – Plenty in my time.

S – *I should stress that this conversation is strictly confidential. When did you last have sex with someone other than your wife?*

P – Two years ago.

S – *At a time when AIDS has had a lot of publicity, you will perhaps not be surprised if I ask whether this was with a man or a woman.*

P – I'm not queer if that's what you mean.

S – *I'm sorry if my question caused offence. May I ask if your difficulty with intercourse is restricted to your wife, or if you have had it with other partners as well?*

Having established that the patient is heterosexual, she is establishing whether his erectile dysfunction affects all relationships (another sign that it is organic as opposed to psychogenic). Having established such a frank discussion, she could now take a more complete history, including age of first sexual experience, range of sexual partners, sexual practices, history of sexually transmitted diseases. Having done so, she summarises the salient points:

S – *So you have had other partners in the past, but only your wife for the last two years. Your interest in sex is as good as it has ever been and you can get an erection but it is not as firm as it should be and you sometimes find it difficult to penetrate. You are finding that you lose your erection quickly and sometimes cannot reach an orgasm or satisfy your wife. Have I understood the situation correctly?*

P – (Nods)

S – *How is this affecting your relationship?*

At this stage, Mary will go on to explore the impact of erectile dysfunction on Mr Hughes and his marriage.

HISTORY SKILLS

> **Core skill: Asking personal details**
>
> 1. Build a rapport with the patient.
>
> 2. Use listening skills to give the patient 'space' to tell their story.
>
> 3. Explain or otherwise 'obtain permission' before asking.
>
> 4. Ask in clear, everyday language.
>
> 5. Use reflection and open questioning to 'draw the patient out'.
>
> 6. Acknowledge embarrassment or other negative emotions.
>
> 7. Respond empathically.
>
> 8. Use open and closed questions to clarify symptoms.
>
> 9. Summarise.

Causes of erectile dysfunction

Having taken a sexual history and established a diagnosis of erectile dysfunction, you should think about underlying causes. These include hypogonadism and, particularly in a diabetic patient, peripheral vascular disease and neuropathy.

- Hypogonadism is relatively rarely the cause of erectile dysfunction. Clues would be a reduced frequency of shaving (loss of 'five o'clock shadow'). Physical examination might reveal small, soft testicles and loss of body hair. Serum testosterone and prolactin should routinely be measured to exclude hypogonadism.
- Intermittent claudication and absent leg pulses would suggest vascular impotence.
- Inappropriate upper body sweating, intermittent diarrhoea and/or vomiting and postural hypotension would suggest autonomic neuropathy and loss of sensation in a stocking sensation would suggest a sensory polyneuropathy.

Management of erectile dysfunction

The first step is to establish whether the patient and his partner wish treatment. They should be offered a joint consultation. Whatever its cause, erectile dysfunction is treated with alprostadil (by intra-cavernosal injection or intra-urethral pellet) or oral sildenafil.

SUGGESTIONS FOR FURTHER PRACTICE

The AIDS epidemic has made it much more acceptable to discuss sex. You should gain confidence in taking sexual histories and learn how to discuss homosexual as well as heterosexual relationships. You may do so when you take general histories. A genitourinary medicine clinic would provide a good opportunity to develop the skill.

HISTORY 7	**Headache**
Level:	**
Setting:	The student is asked to interview a middle-aged female standardised patient; the examiner observes
Time:	10 min

TASK

E – *Please take a history from this lady and then present it to me.*

RESPONSE

As you read through the following dialogue, consider the student's performance carefully. You may wish to write a structured critique and think what you would do differently before reading our critique.

S – *Good morning. My name is Tracy. I'm a fourth year medical student. I'd like to take a history; that's all right isn't it. How old are you?*

P – 52.

S – *What is your job?*

P – I'm just a housewife.

S – *How many children do you have?*

P – None. We weren't able to have any.

S – *What symptoms have you got?*

P – I've got this terrible headache.

S – *What sort of pain is it?*

P – It isn't what you'd call a pain; it's as though my head's going to burst.

S – *Where is the pain?*

P – That's rather difficult to answer. My whole head feels –

S – *How long have you had it?*

P – About 6 months.

S – *Is there anything that makes the headache worse?*

P – Not that I'm aware of.

S – *Is there anything you can do that takes the pain away?*

P – I've been taking a lot of codeine tablets. I'm a bit concerned about that because I've heard that too much codeine can be harmful.

S – *Does anything other than codeine relieve the pain?*

P – I haven't found anything else that works.

S – *Do you have any other symptoms associated with the pain?*

P – I don't think so.

S – *What previous illnesses have you had?*

P – The usual childhood ones; and a hysterectomy.

S – *Have you ever had TB, diabetes or jaundice?*

P – No.

S – *Are there any illnesses which run through your family?*

P – My mother died of cancer of the neck of the womb; she was just 45.

S – *What did your father die from?*

P – Old age. He died last year.

S – *How old was he when he died?*

P – 86.

S – *Do you have any brothers or sisters?*

P – Just an older brother in Australia but I'm not in contact with him. He didn't even come to my father's funeral.

S – *So you don't know if he has any illnesses.*

P – I suppose not.

S – *What does your husband do?*

P – He's on the sick.

S – *Do you have any financial worries?*

P – Obviously we do, with neither of us working.

S – *What sort of house do you live in?*

P – A council house; why?

S – *Just a routine question. Do you smoke?*

P – Yes.

S – *How much?*

P – Twenty a day.

S – *How much do you drink?*

P – We can't afford to drink.

S – *Are you on any tablets other than codeine?*

P – No.

S – *Have you had any fits, faints or blackouts?*

P – No.

S – *Have you had any weakness, loss of sensation, unsteadiness, dizziness, or trouble with your eyes or ears?*

P – No.

S – *Any breathlessness, cough, chest pain or ankle swelling?*

P – No.

S – *Any problems with your waterworks?*

P – No.

S – *Any abdominal pain, vomiting or diarrhoea?*

P – No.

Silence; student turns to examiner.

E – *Could you now present the history to me?*

S – *She is a 52-year-old married housewife with no children who has a 6-month history of headache. It is a bursting feeling and affects her whole head. It doesn't radiate anywhere and there are no precipitating or relieving factors. She had the usual childhood illnesses and a hysterectomy but has never had TB, diabetes or jaundice. Her father died of old age and her mother of ca cervix. She has one brother who is well, as far as she knows. She has no children and there*

45

is no other family history. She smokes 20 cigarettes per day but does not drink. Her husband is unemployed and they have money problems. She only takes codeine tablets. On systems review, she does not admit to any fits, faints, blackouts and there's nothing else in the CNS, and no symptoms in the GUS, RS, CVS or GIS.

E – *What do you think is wrong with her?*

S – *Ummm. Could she have a tension headache?*

Critique

This dialogue is the stuff of examination failure. You may think it is a ridiculous pastiche but how many similar mistakes do you make under stress? You might argue that the student took a history 'by the books' and should get credit for it but that is precisely where she went wrong. An examiner would take a very dim view of her rigid, interrogative style, and the way she concentrated on facts to the exclusion of emotional content, was completely insensitive when the patient showed annoyance, and did not explore the symptoms with any intelligence or understanding. Here is a more detailed critique of her performance:

Communication

- **Introductions:** did not ask the patient's name and made no effort to put her at ease.
- **Consent:** asked permission to interview in a way that gave the patient no choice.
- **Listening skills:** showed no sensitivity to the patient's view, translated her words into medical ones inaccurately and made no attempt to check that she had 'heard' correctly.
- **Verbal skills:**
  - **Question-framing:** almost exclusively used closed questions and strung multiple questions together.
  - **Verbal facilitation:** did not clarify the information volunteered by the patient and interrupted what might have been a useful clarification.
  - **Use of language:** used medical language inappropriately and made little effective use of lay language.
  - **Explaining:** did not explain why questions were being asked.
- **Emotional content:** ignored it completely, and missed one after another important cue.
- **Summarisation:** did not summarise at all.
- **Factual content:** obtained an incomplete description of the problem, framed largely in the interviewer's terms.
- **Patient's perceptions and concerns:** did not identify them at all.
- **Ending:** did not acknowledge the patient's contribution, invite any additional comments or questions; in fact, did not wind up the interview at all.

Interview structure

46

The student used the medical history structure as a 'straitjacket' rather than a broad framework within which to hear the patient's story. Some sections, such as 'social history', showed that she did not clearly understand their purpose.

Content

The student followed a learned series of questions about 'a pain'. She, herself, came up with none that were diagnostically useful and did not follow clues that were offered her. An examiner would have to conclude from her questioning that, as well as having seriously defective communication skills, she did not know much about the causes of headache or the features which distinguish them (see 'Diagnosis of headache' later). An intelligent approach would have been to cover the following features:

- Any prodromal symptoms
- A clear description of the headache
- Its site(s) and radiation
- Its timing through the day, and history
- Any associated symptoms
- Precipitants and causes
- Relevant negatives
- Relevant psycho-social details
- The patient's perceptions and concerns.

She could then have constructed a differential diagnosis based on the information obtained and the facts in Table 3.3 below, and said which diagnoses were most likely.

Presentation

She regurgitated facts without showing that she had understood them. She offered no differential diagnosis, and no suggestions about what she would do next. She was flawed when asked to interpret the history and did not even seem to be expecting the question.

Standardised patient script

To give you insight into the way exams are set up, here is a script which might have been given to the standardised patient in the interview above. It illustrates just how badly the student mishandled this station.

> You have always been a worrier and prone to headaches. You had to take time away from school due to headaches after the death of your mother from cancer of the cervix at the age of 45. You are infertile and have no children. This has been a major disappointment to both you and your husband, and he blames you for it. You have lost touch with your one brother who emigrated to Australia when you were still a teenager. You were very close to your father and his death last year at the age of 86 hit you hard. At first, you put a brave face on it but your husband's redundancy soon afterwards created stress at home and made it harder to cope with your bereavement.

> For the last 6 months, the headaches have returned, they are worse than they have ever been and you are having one every day. You experience it as a bursting sensation that is worse towards the end of the day. Sometimes you get

Table 3.3 Features which distinguish some important causes of headache

	Tension	Classical migraine	Cervical spondylosis	Raised intracranial pressure	Cranial arteritis
Prodrome	None	Visual aura	None	None	None
Nature	May be 'band-like', or dull ache, sometimes with sharp exacerbations	May be throbbing. Variable intensity; may be very severe	May be described as 'ache'	May be dull, throbbing	Varies in severity
Site	Typically biparietal, bifrontal or over vertex. Pain may be located to scalp rather than 'inside head'	May be generalised or localised	Occipital radiating over vertex	May be whole head or localised	Frontal and/or occipital. May be associated with jaw pain (on mastication)
Timing through day	Often day-long, worsening towards evening	No distinctive pattern	No distinctive pattern	Intermittent in the early stages Typically present on waking and may improve through the day	No distinctive pattern
History	May have developed or worsened shortly before presentation; careful questioning may reveal long history	May date back to childhood; attacks may have been very infrequent. Attacks may 'cluster' over days or weeks with periods of freedom. History often erratic and unpredictable	Onset later in life	Recent onset, worsening	Recent onset

Table 3.3 (cont'd)

	Tension	Classical migraine	Cervical spondylosis	Raised intracranial pressure	Cranial arteritis
Associated symptoms	May be fullness in the head, dizziness, extreme tiredness or other somatic symptoms	Photophobia, nausea, vomiting	Neck pain	Patient 'ill', often with other neurological symptoms. Vomiting	Soreness of scalp, particularly temporal region. Visual disturbances. Systemic malaise. Stiffness of shoulders and/or hips
Precipitant or cause	May be an identifiable cause of tension (e.g. work or family stress) but often not	May be related to foods, stress, tiredness (though may occur when relaxing), contraceptive pill	Head movement	Made worse by coughing or stooping	None

an intolerable feeling of pressure on top of your head. You have not noticed anything that brings the headache on; only codeine relieves it but it is making you constipated and you are worried that you might become addicted to it. You have no symptoms in your eyes either before the headaches or during them. You are generally lacking in energy and your mood is low, but you have not noticed any other specific symptoms.

You know someone who died of a brain tumour after the doctor dismissed his headaches as unimportant and referred him late for a brain scan. You are worried that you may have a tumour and would like a scan for reassurance.

Diagnosis of headache

Table 3.3 shows some common causes of headache and the characteristics that distinguish them. A skilled interviewer would encourage the patient to describe the symptoms and use good communication skills both to communicate empathy and obtain important psycho-social details which the patient might be reluctant to divulge.

SUGGESTIONS FOR FURTHER PRACTICE

Headache is a common symptom. Every medical ward has at least one patient suffering from it, it is one of the commonest causes of general medical out-patient referral, it is a bread-and-butter problem in neurology clinics and general practitioners manage it every day of the week. There is no shortage of opportunities to practise the skill; if you feel unsure of your ability, seek out an opportunity to take a history and ask a doctor to 'debrief' you on it.

HISTORY 8	**Collapse**
Level:	***
Setting:	The student is asked to interview a 'real' patient observed by an examiner seated in a corner
Time:	10 min

TASK

E – *Good morning. I am Dr Brain. This is Mrs Forest. She was referred to my outpatient clinic last Friday. Please take up to 10 minutes to obtain her history. I will then ask you questions about her for 5 minutes. I will sit here and observe you taking the history but please try to ignore me as much as you can.*

RESPONSE

Student shakes hands with the patient.

S – *Good morning. My name is Tom. I am a final year medical student. May I interview you?*

P – Yes, you go ahead, ask me anything you want. After all, I'm stuck here; nothing better to do with my time.

S – *As you have heard, we have up to 10 minutes. During that time, I would like to hear what it was that brought you to see Dr Brain. I may need to ask you quite a lot of questions. I hope you won't mind that. Please tell me at once if any of my questions bother you. Will you tell me your age and say just a few words about yourself?*

P – I'm 55. What else do you want to know? I work in a newsagent, I've got a dog and three cats, I've been married for 30 years and he's been on the sick for 15 of them and the doctor said I had to come and see him (nods to Dr Brain) to be checked out. I think it's a lot of fuss about nothing. It was the heat and all the going-on with the woman next door. If you ask me, they should be kicked out, these scroungers – never done an honest day's work in their lives, and him, sitting on his backside watching the TV all the time when there's bills to be paid …

S – *It sounds as though there is a lot going on in your life and I hope you'll tell me more in a moment or two but what were you saying about the heat?*

P – Well it's no surprise, is it, when you're on your feet all day and it gets that hot in there, it's bound to upset your hormones …

S – *Upset your hormones?*

P – Well it is, isn't it? It's bound to …

S – *I'd like to answer your question, but I need a little help from you first. It sounds as though something happened on a hot day when you'd been on your feet for a long time. Please tell me what happened.*

P – Like I said, it was nothing really. You'd expect it at my age. And I told him not to

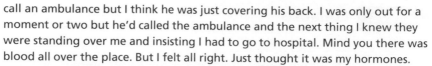

call an ambulance but I think he was just covering his back. I was only out for a moment or two but he'd called the ambulance and the next thing I knew they were standing over me and insisting I had to go to hospital. Mind you there was blood all over the place. But I felt all right. Just thought it was my hormones.

S – *It sounds as though you had a frightening experience.*

P – You're telling me. Finding yourself on the floor with all the customers gawping down at you. Thinking all sorts of things.

S – *All sorts of things?*

P – Well he said it probably wouldn't happen again.

S – *Happen again?*

P – That time it happened before.

S – *Happened before?*

P – Like I said, he said it likely as not wouldn't happen again.

S – *Thank you for telling me so much about your experiences, Mrs Forest. There are so many important things in what you have said that I would like to repeat them back to you so you can tell me if I have understood them correctly. On a hot day, after you had been on your feet for a long time, it sounds as though you lost consciousness and collapsed to the ground. You came round on the floor. There was blood all over the place so you must have hurt yourself. You were surrounded by people looking down at you. An ambulance was called and you were taken to hospital. It was an alarming experience for you. It sounds as though something similar has happened before and one of the worst things for you is that you had hoped it would never happen again. In a moment, I'm sure you'll tell me if I've understood you correctly but it would help me very much if you could describe what happened on that day. Please start from the moment you knew something was up.*

P – Like I said, it was a hot day and we'd been rushed off our feet all morning. It was that smell .. and I felt horrible … and next thing I knew there they all were gawping at me.

S – *Can you describe the smell and the horrible feeling?*

P – It was like burnt rubber, that smell, and I just felt something was going to happen.

S – *And how did you feel when you came round?*

P – I just felt horrible, really strange, as though I wasn't really there.

S – *Do you remember falling?*

P – No.

S – *Did you bite your tongue or wet yourself?*

P – My tongue was really sore afterwards.

S – *Can we now come back to that other time it happened. <u>What</u> happened?*

P – It was that smell, and feeling something was going to happen. But they didn't take me to hospital.

S – *Did you lose consciousness on that other occasion?*

P – I was down on the ground, if that's what you mean. Don't remember much more about it.

S – *And have there been other occasions?*

P – You're as bad as the rest of them. He kept going on about it after that time in the Isle of Wight, but it's all right for him, sitting on the settee all day watching

television. If he had to work as hard as I do to pay the bills, maybe he'd have his off days too.

Critique

Taking a history from a talkative patient is a challenge to any professional, particularly when time is tight. Far from losing him marks, Tom's expert handling of Mrs Forest's talkativeness will have scored highly. If the dialogue had continued, it is likely that he would have got into more and more technical detail and he paced the interview well enough to accomplish his task in the allotted time. His skill was to turn a rambling narrative into a clear and informative history. This station illustrates the following points:

1. The process of good communication.
2. The structure of the interview.
3. A systematic approach to interviewing a patient with 'collapse'.

Communication skills
The skills in this interview were:

- Not being flustered by an unpromising start.
- Being very courteous and using that courtesy to keep Mrs Forest 'to task'.
- Recognising Mrs Forest's anxiety and reflecting the emotional content of what she said back to her. Her talkativeness may have been a 'smoke screen' to cover her anxiety so his acknowledgement of her anxiety helped him get quickly to the 'meat' of the diagnostic history. She will have found him a sympathetic, 'listening' interviewer.
- Obtaining consent, not just to take the history but to get into detailed questioning where necessary
- His questioning strategy: making good use of open questions, echoing Mrs Forest's words to steer her into talking about things which he thought were important, and delaying very closed questions until Mrs Forest had been given ample opportunity to get things off her chest.

Above all, his interview was efficient and effective because he used communication skills to obtain a very full history and simultaneously show empathy to the patient.

Interview structure
This dialogue illustrates the value of not imposing too rigid a structure on an interview. What might have been dismissed as talkativeness gave rich information about the psycho-social background of the patient simultaneously with information about the presenting complaint. An interviewer who only had ears for the presenting complaint might have lost her cooperation by showing lack of concern, and wasted time because all the psycho-social details would have to be extracted less efficiently by closed questioning later on. The challenge is to take in details of more than one component of the medical history at once. The

introduction to this section suggests how you can take notes in a way that turns a disorganised history into an organised presentation (page 25).

Approach to a patient with 'collapse'

The term 'collapse' refers to a short-lived mishap without permanent physical sequelae. Since patients are usually seen after the event and physical examination is often normal, diagnosis hinges almost entirely on good history-taking. First, distinguish between dysfunction of the central nervous system and a mechanical fall. Second, distinguish between the two main causes of brain dysfunction: SYNCOPE (transient reduction of cerebral blood flow) and EPILEPSY. Third, consider other possible causes such as some metabolic disturbance (e.g. hypoglycaemia), drug effect or intoxication. That is done by obtaining an extremely detailed description of:

- The circumstances in which the collapse happened
- Any prodromal symptoms
- Whether the patient lost consciousness
- The last thing they remember before doing so
- The next thing they remember
- How they felt after (or during) the attack
- Whether they bit their tongue, were incontinent or were noted to be stiff, shaking or frothing at the mouth
- Any other attacks and their similarity to the present one
- Risk factors, including personal and family history.

A full discussion of the differential diagnosis of collapse is beyond the scope of this book but should be second nature to a student by qualification.

Core skill: Responding to a patient's talkativeness

1. Do not abandon your listening skills; the more you try to interrupt, the more the patient will want to have their say.

2. Wait for a natural break, then reflect back an important point in the patient's narrative.

3. Recognise talkativeness as a possible defence mechanism; recognise and respond empathically to the emotional content of the history.

4. 'Steer' the patient by selectively reflecting, paraphrasing and summarising aspects of the narrative.

5. Accept that the information will not come as concisely as you would like and avoid resorting to closed questions, at least until you have developed a rapport and hear the patient's story.

6. Accept that the history will not come out in the order that you would choose but take orderly notes (page 25).

7. Remain calm and courteous.

SUGGESTIONS FOR FURTHER PRACTICE

The ability to interview talkative patients in limited time is a key skill for clinical examinations. There is no shortage of people with a lot to say on wards, in clinics and general practice surgeries so seek them out. Practise directing the flow of their discourse, whilst listening intently, and focussing what they have to say into a 'history'.

HISTORY 9	**Skin rash**
Level:	**
Setting:	OSCE station; structured viva
Time:	5 min

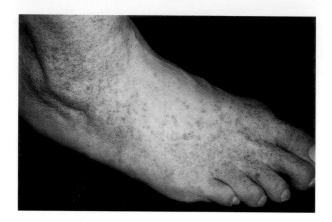

TASK

E – (Shows you the above photograph.) *A 16-year-old boy is brought to the General Practitioner's surgery because of a skin rash like the one shown in this photograph. It came on abruptly 48 hours ago. The lesions are macular and do not blanch on pressure. He is apyrexial and felt well enough to go to school today. What points would you cover in the history?*

RESPONSE

Meningococcal disease has received so much publicity that you might be tempted to orientate your history towards it; however, the diagnosis is most unlikely on the grounds that:

- He remains well despite having had the rash for 48 h; he would be lucky to survive untreated meningococcal septicaemia for that length of time.
- He is apyrexial.
- The petechial appearance in this photograph is not typical of meningococcal disease.

You could indicate to the examiner, in a few words, why meningococcal septicaemia is an unlikely diagnosis in this case.

Petechial lesions are strongly suggestive of haemorrhage at the capillary level due either to **disease of the capillary wall** (e.g. Henoch–Schönlein purpura) or **thrombocytopenia**. Thrombocytopenia is commoner and a more likely diagnosis than Henoch–Schönlein purpura in an otherwise well person, but bear the other possibility in mind.

Next, think logically through the causes of thrombocytopenia. They are:

1. Decreased production of platelets:
   - Aplastic anaemia
   - Leukaemia, lymphoma or other neoplastic disease affecting the bone marrow
   - Myelosuppressive drugs or irradiation
   - Megaloloblastic anaemia.
2. Increased platelet destruction:
   - Immune:
     Idiopathic thrombocytopenia
     Drug-induced
   - Associated with vasculitis.

Table 3.4 suggests how you could tailor your history to explore those possible causes.

One way of impressing the examiner is to ask pertinent and focussed questions relatively early in the history. In particular, don't wait too long to ask questions that are immediately relevant to the presenting symptom. In the present case, purpura strongly suggests haematological disease so it makes sense to ask the haematological questions of the systems review after you have heard the history of the presenting complaint; positive answers will focus your enquiries and help you make best use of limited time.

SUGGESTIONS FOR FURTHER PRACTICE

Make sure that you are able to recognise a petechial rash and discuss the differential diagnosis fluently. It is a relatively common skin manifestation of systemic disease, and one that any competent practitioner must be able to recognise. Remind yourself of the symptoms of red cell and white cell disease. Think out how you would have responded if the 'trigger' had been a blood count showing neutropenia or anaemia.

Table 3.4 How to tailor a history to the differential diagnosis of thrombocytopenia

History of presenting complaint	Listen carefully for any symptoms or illness preceding the appearance of purpura that might suggest systemic disease. Ask specifically about: • Malaise • Weight loss • Febrile symptoms Ask about other haematological symptoms that might suggest bone marrow disease: • Platelets: Evidence of bleeding (maloena, haematuria, haemoptysis etc.) • Red cells: Symptoms of anaemia (ankle swelling, breathlessness) • White cells: Increased susceptibility to infection Ask specifically whether the onset of purpura was preceded by a viral or other infection. Acute idiopathic thrombocytopenia in young adults follows an acute infection in over a half of cases
Previous medical history	Enquire specifically about: • Previous haematological disease • Episodes of purpura
Family history	Enquire about: • Any haematological disease • Pernicious anaemia or other organ-specific autoimmune disease
Social history	Enquire about: • Hobbies or other activities which might involve exposure to drugs or toxins • Substance abuse • Radiation exposure
Drug history	Take a careful drug history, including non-prescription drugs

Systems review	Enquire specifically about:
	• GIS:
	    Abdominal pain (Typically present in Henoch–Schönlein purpura)
	    Symptoms of malabsorption that might be associated with B_{12} or folate deficiency
	• MSS:
	    Arthralgia (Again, typically present in Henoch–Schönlein purpura)
	• Skin:
	    Pruritis (May occur in lymphoma)

HISTORY 10	**Thirst and polyuria**
Level:	**
Setting:	A middle-aged standardised patient
Time:	10 min

TASK

E – (Hands you a referral letter from a GP to the hospital.) *You are a hospital doctor who has received this referral letter. Please interview the patient and see what you think the diagnosis might be.*

> Dear Doctor,
>
> Mr Jones was brought to the surgery by his wife, who complains that he is constantly drinking water, tea and anything he can lay his hands on. He goes to the toilet hourly during the day and gets up three times at night. He makes light of this problem and hasn't come to the surgery for over 20 years.
>
> Please see and advise.
>
> Yours sincerely,
>
> Dr George Pea

RESPONSE

Although this is a history station, the examiner has given you unusually clear direction about how to approach it. The instruction suggests you should be quite focussed in your history-taking and concentrate on the differential diagnosis. However, do not be so focussed that you abandon the communication skills described in History Station 1: Chest pain.

Diagnostic logic

The causes of polyuria and polydipsia in rough order of frequency are:

- Habitual excessive drinking ('hysterical polydipsia')
- Diabetes mellitus
- Chronic renal failure causing nephrogenic diabetes insipidus
- Hypercalcaemia or severe, chronic hypokalaemia
- Cranial diabetes insipidus.

Hysterical polydipsia is very much a diagnosis of exclusion. Although you must work logically through the physical causes, be alert to any hints of psychological problems or psychiatric disease. A reasonable approach would be to:

1. Use your usual approach (History Station 1: Chest pain) to obtain the patient's description of the presenting complaint.
2. Ask specific questions that would support the diagnoses above:
   - Weight loss, lethargy, balanitis, blurred vision and/or a positive family history would support a diagnosis of diabetes mellitus
   - A history of renal disease and symptoms of uraemia – e.g. itching of the skin – would support chronic renal failure
   - Abdominal pain, constipation and weight loss would support hypercalcaemia; severe hypokalaemia might cause muscle weakness
   - Headaches, lethargy, weight loss and impotence might suggest hypopituitarism associated with cranial diabetes insipidus.
3. Obtain a drug history and previous medical history.
4. Enquire about personal and psychological factors that might be associated with hysterical polydipsia.

E – *This investigation was performed on Mr Jones; what is it, what does it show and how does that help your diagnosis?*

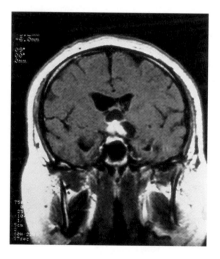

This is an MR scan showing a mass in the region of the hypothalamus. You would not be expected to know this but, taken together with symptoms suggestive of diabetes insipidus, the likely diagnosis is a craniopharyngioma.

E – *Having seen the result of that investigation, how would you now investigate Mr Jones' thirst and polyuria?*

The following investigations would support a diagnosis of diabetes insipidus:

- Normal fasting plasma glucose, serum calcium, potassium, urea and creatinine, excluding the other diagnoses listed above
- A urine volume over 3 L in a 24-h collection
- A low urine osmolality in the presence of a high plasma osmolality
- A high plasma sodium concentration (this *may* be found in diabetes insipidus but the patient is extremely dehydrated by the time it occurs)
- During a water deprivation test, the patient continues to pass dilute urine despite not drinking and the plasma osmolality rises.

SUGGESTIONS FOR FURTHER PRACTICE

Become familiar with the appearance of cranial CT and MR scans so that you can easily spot gross abnormalities; it is unlikely that you would be presented with subtle ones in an undergraduate examination.

HISTORY SKILLS

HISTORY 11	**Back pain**
Level:	**
Setting:	A male standardised patient
Time:	10 min

TASK

E – (Hands you a radiology report.) *Mr Thomas consulted another doctor a week ago with back pain who arranged a radiograph, of which this is the report. Please take a history.*

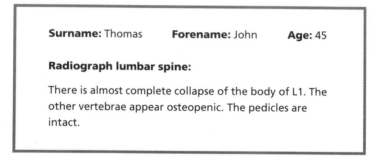

Surname: Thomas **Forename:** John **Age:** 45

Radiograph lumbar spine:

There is almost complete collapse of the body of L1. The other vertebrae appear osteopenic. The pedicles are intact.

RESPONSE

The radiograph has shown a serious abnormality that needs to be fully explored. The weakest response would be to take an unfocussed general history. Second best would be to concentrate just on the history of the back pain or on pointers to underlying malignant disease. The optimum approach is to strike a balance between:

1. Obtaining full details of the back pain
2. Enquiring about possible complications of vertebral collapse
3. Going very thoroughly into possible underlying causes.

Back pain

The history should include a detailed description of the time course and nature of the symptoms. Did any trauma precede the back pain? Remember that epileptic fits can cause enough compression force in the spine to crush a vertebra.

Complications of vertebral collapse

This may cause nerve root entrapment and/or spinal cord compression. You should ask if the pain radiates in the L1 distribution; if bladder and bowel function and/or sensation are affected; and if muscle power and sensation in the legs is abnormal.

Causes

Your history should seek evidence of the diseases that can cause generalised osteopenia:

1. Osteoporosis
2. Malignant disease
3. Hyperparathyroidism.

Osteoporosis

Ostepoporosis of this severity is unusual in a young man. It could be caused by:

- Severe and longstanding hypogonadism (e.g. Klinefelter's syndrome not treated with testosterone replacement therapy)
- Endocrine disease such as Cushing's syndrome or thyrotoxicosis
- Immobility
- Severe chronic illness or malnutrition.

Enquire about systemic disease, immobility and endocrine disease. Ask quite specifically about symptoms of male sexual function, as described in History 6: Erectile dysfunction. It is not unknown for patients to be completely unaware that they have been hypogonadal throughout adult life because they have never known differently.

Malignant disease

Multiple myeloma or metastatic malignancy can cause diffuse (as well as focal) bone loss and mimic osteoporosis. Malignancy would be the likely diagnosis if there were erosion of the pedicles but intact pedicles argue against it. Enquire about symptoms affecting any system that might suggest malignant disease.

Hyperparathyroidism

Hyperparathyroidism can cause diffuse bone loss. Were that the diagnosis, Mr Thomas would be hypercalcaemic and his symptoms might include:

- Apathy
- Weight loss
- Anorexia
- Thirst
- Polyuria
- Dyspepsia
- Abdominal pain
- A history of hypertension
- Symptoms of renal stone.

There might also be a family history of hyperparathyroidism.

As you go through his previous medical history, family history, social history, drug history and systems review, be alert for any risk factors for the diseases listed above, and any evidence to suggest that Mr Thomas has one of them.

SUGGESTIONS FOR FURTHER PRACTICE

Remind yourself of the malignancies that most commonly metastasise to bone and think what symptoms would suggest those diagnoses. Revise multiple myeloma; think how you might recognise it in the history and examination, and what investigations you would do.

HISTORY SKILLS

HISTORY 12 Pyrexia

Level:	*
Setting:	You are interviewed by an examiner
Time:	5 min

TASK

E – *A 67-year-old woman has 'gone off her legs'. She has a temperature of 38°C and is lying with the blankets firmly pulled up around her neck. What points would you cover in the history?*

RESPONSE

This station should be read in conjunction with History 4: Diarrhoea, which describes how the medical history structure can be applied in a 'problem-orientated' way to a symptom/sign that has many possible causes. Your history should cover:

Presenting history

1. Symptoms of fever:
   - Feeling cold
   - Shivering
   - Shaking; the term 'rigor' describes a severe shaking attack.
2. Any symptoms that point to a viral illness: *I'm aching all over and my nose is running.*
3. Symptoms referrable to the individual systems:
   - Frequency, dysuria, haematuria, pain in the loin or supra-pubic region
   - Chest pain, dyspnoea, cough, sputum production, wheeze
   - Headache, photophobia, neck pain or stiffness
   - Abdominal pain, vomiting, change in bowel habit, jaundice or a change in the colour of urine and/or motions.

Previous history

Any previous medical history, including surgery and accidents, could be relevant. Careful exploration could uncover a relevant problem such as rheumatic fever in childhood (which left the patient with a heart valve at risk of bacterial endocarditis) or a kidney stone predisposing to urinary infection. Enquire specifically about recent medical contacts or problems for which the patient did not consult a doctor. Ask about influenza immunisation.

Social history

Enquire about travel, contact with another person with an infectious disease, or the possibility of having eaten contaminated food.

HISTORY SKILLS

Drug history

Take a detailed history of prescription and non-prescription drugs, particularly antibiotics. Take a detailed smoking and alcohol history, remembering that smoking increases the risk of chest infections and alcohol abuse predisposes to many diseases, including peritonitis and septicaemia.

Systems review

This is a chance to pick up any symptoms not discovered in your questioning about the presenting problem. You should have developed a battery of screening questions that are likely to pick up dysfunction of the individual systems.

E – *Having taken the history and examined the patient, you have still not been able to make a diagnosis. What investigations would you do?*

- Full blood count: a neutrophil leucocytosis would suggest bacterial infection
- Blood culture: to diagnose septicaemia
- Chest radiograph: may show pulmonary infiltrates diagnostic of pneumonia even when there are no diagnostic symptoms or signs
- Urine microscopy and culture: urinary infection is a common cause of 'PUO' in older people.

SUGGESTIONS FOR FURTHER PRACTICE

Draw up a list of 10 (or more) causes of fever. Test yourself out on their characteristic symptoms and signs and the most informative investigations.

HISTORY 13 Lethargy

Level:	*
Setting:	A 63-year-old male simulated patient
Time:	5 min

TASK

E – *Please take a history from this patient.*
When asked what is troubling him, the patient replies: *I'm absolutely tired out, doctor.*

RESPONSE

An epidemiologist is said to have shown that 80% of the general population suffer from tiredness and the remaining 20% suffer from total exhaustion. You do not yet have evidence that there is anything medically wrong with the patient. The thing *not* to do is to launch into a battery of closed questions. You need a better description of:

1. What the patient is experiencing.
2. How it is affecting him.

And you need to consider

3. What might be the cause.

Presenting complaint

Patients who feel tired often fear that there is something seriously wrong with them. They may be very suggestible. Closed questioning tends to produce a lot of non-specific positive responses that take a lot of time to follow through so, as in almost every situation, you need to obtain a history in the patient's own words as far as possible. If you are not sure how to do that, re-read the introduction to this section and History 1: Chest pain. If you want to be reminded of the dangers of excessive closed questioning, read History 7: Headache.

What the patient is experiencing
'Tiredness' may mean:

- Non-specific malaise
- A change in the pattern of sleep: increased or altered hours of sleep or a tendency to sleep during the daytime
- Lack of drive and motivation
- Physical weakness.

67

How it is affecting him

Tiredness should be taken more seriously if it affects the patient's activities. A subjective feeling of lack of energy that does not interfere with work or social life is less significant than one that has caused the person to change job or give up a hobby. Even if the tiredness turns out to be the Chronic Fatigue Syndrome (CFS), a benign condition, you need to assess the functional disability that it causes.

The cause

As you go through the history, you are attempting to distinguish between:

- The sort of tiredness any of us might get
- Tiredness as a manifestation of a psycho-social problem; e.g. alcohol abuse or marital disharmony
- Tiredness due to disease.

Loss of weight or the presence of other systemic symptoms makes it much more likely that tiredness is 'significant'. You have little time so you need to make focussed enquiries into each of the 'compartments' of the medical history.

Previous medical history

Ask about any previous illness or chronic disease that might be affecting the patient now, including psychiatric disease.

Family history

Ask about diabetes and other autoimmune diseases, or anything else that runs strongly through the family.

Social history

Apart from establishing the severity of the tiredness, as described above, probe into any psycho-social factors that might be making the patient feel low; e.g. threat of unemployment, illness in a close relative. You might ask a question such as: *Is there anything in your personal life which might be affecting the way you feel, or taking the edge off your enjoyment of life?*

Drug and alcohol history

Enquire about any prescription or non-prescription drugs (e.g. beta blockers, which commonly cause tiredness), alcohol (History 14: Alcohol history) and, if time permits and the circumstances suggest that it is appropriate, substance or drug abuse.

Systems review

Your best chance of finding a cause of tiredness comes from identifying associated

Table 3.5 Examples of symptoms which, associated with tiredness, could point to particular diagnoses

	Cardiovascular	Respiratory	Gastrointestinal	Genitourinary	Neurological	Psychiatric	Haematological	Endocrine/ Metabolic	Infection
Symptoms	Dyspnoea Cough Ankle swelling	Dyspnoea Cough Weight loss Haemoptysis	Diarrhoea Abdominal pain Rectal bleeding Weight loss	Abdominal pain Fever Haematuria	Headache Increased eating Personality change	Sleep disturbance Low mood Tearfulness Loss of pleasure and purpose	Breathlessness Blood loss	Polyuria Polydipsia Blurred vision Balanitis/ pruritis vulvae Weight loss	Sore throat Enlarged lymph glands
Diagnosis	Heart failure	Carcinoma of the bronchus TB	Inflammatory bowel disease	Renal carcinoma	Hypothalamic tumour	Depression	Anaemia	Diabetes mellitus	Infectious mononucleosis

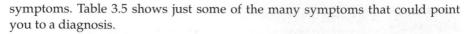

symptoms. Table 3.5 shows just some of the many symptoms that could point you to a diagnosis.

More often than not, no cause is found for profound tiredness and the diagnosis is CFS. This term is used to describe a common, debilitating condition of unknown cause that may drag on for months or years. When you come to the end of presenting your history, you will score well if you offer a broad differential diagnosis and include CFS in it, unless there is a pointer in the history to some other underlying disease.

SUGGESTIONS FOR FURTHER PRACTICE

Try the same approach to another non-specific symptom such as weight loss or weight gain. Think out a differential diagnosis, and then think how you would set about taking the history. Develop your history-taking skills by trying to obtain a clear and detailed history from patients with non-specific symptoms. Like headache (History 7) there is no shortage of patients on whom to practise this skill.

HISTORY 14 | Alcohol history

Level:	**
Setting:	A 48-year-old male simulated patient. The examiner observes and rates you
Time:	5 min

TASK

E – *You are a general practitioner. Mr Stewart has seen one of your partners complaining of tiredness. His liver function tests have come back grossly abnormal with a gamma glutamyl transferase level six times the upper limit of normal. His MCV is also raised at 110 fl. Please take an alcohol history.*

RESPONSE

This station tests knowledge of alcohol abuse and its effects as well as your interviewing skill.

Interviewing skill

There are close parallels between this station and History 6: Erectile dysfunction. Both take you into what may be very sensitive territory. See Core skill: Asking personal details, page 42, for general guidance.

One way to start would be with a narrative introduction, such as: *You saw my colleague recently and he checked your blood count and a test of your liver. Both are abnormal. That could happen if you were drinking more alcohol than is good for you. May I ask you some questions about your drinking habits?* Patients who abuse alcohol may be evasive in their answers. Watch out for the person who replies in very vague and general terms. Mr Stewart's GGT and MCV are grossly abnormal and give you strong grounds to suspect alcohol abuse. This is a time to be persistent and very specific in your questioning, for example: *I am still finding it difficult to build up a very clear picture of the amount you drink. Will you take me through exactly what you drank yesterday?*

The core skill box lists the components of a thorough alcohol history. The examiner will expect you to cover these including the simple CAGE questionnaire.

> #### Core skill: Taking an alcohol history
>
> Your history should cover:
>
> 1. His alcohol intake.
>   - How much alcohol he drinks in a typical week
>   - What different types of alcohol he drinks

Core skill: *(cont'd)*

- Where he drinks, and whether he drinks alone or in company
- Whether his drinking habit is consistent or he drinks in sprees.

2. Risk factors for alcohol abuse; e.g. working as a licensee.

3. Features of alcohol dependence:
   - Whether he is aware of a compulsion to drink
   - Whether his tolerance of alcohol is increased; i.e. drinks heavily without feeling or appearing drunk
   - Withdrawal symptoms:
     - Typically first thing in the morning or after periods of abstinence
     - Symptoms include shaking, agitation, nausea, retching and sweating
     - Symptoms are relieved by drinking alcohol
   - Hallucinations or altered perceptions
   - History of drinking in the morning, or at other times to relieve symptoms.

4. Social effects:
   - Marital disharmony, divorce or family stress
   - Poor job performance or unemployment
   - Convictions for driving under the influence of alcohol or other offences
   - Financial problems

5. Previous management:
   - Attempts to stop drinking
   - Detoxification.

6. Health complications:
   - Peptic ulceration or dyspepsia
   - History of pancreatitis
   - Hypertension
   - Ischaemic heart disease
   - Heart failure due to alcoholic cardiomyopathy
   - Liver disease or haematemesis due to portal hypertension
   - Anaemia
   - Peripheral neuropathy, ataxia
   - Amnesia or other cognitive dysfunction
   - Epilepsy
   - Depression or anxiety
   - Accidents.

7. The CAGE questionnaire:
   - A patient who answers yes to three or four of the following four questions is very likely to be dependent on alcohol:
     - Have you ever tried to Cut down your drinking?
     - Do you ever get Angry when people talk to you about your drinking?
     - Do you ever feel Guilty about your drinking?
     - Do you ever take an 'Eye opener'?

SUGGESTIONS FOR FURTHER PRACTICE

It is estimated that at least a quarter of patients on general medical wards are there because of alcohol abuse and that there is one unrecognised case for every one that is recognised so there is no shortage of opportunity to practise taking an alcohol history. In doing so, use your listening skills to encourage patients to take you into their confidence, and explore the many facets of alcohol dependence listed above.

CHAPTER 4

Examination skills

Introduction

Within OSCEs, you will always be tested on your ability to examine body systems. The complexity of the stations is dependent on your seniority. In the initial stages, the stations will test your ability simply to *demonstrate* a skill. As you approach the final examination (and beyond) the OSCE will require you to elicit physical signs, determine what is abnormal, interpret the pattern of abnormality and reach a diagnosis.

BASIC LEVEL

The stations are characteristically short (e.g. 5 min) and confined to demonstrating examination sequence for a body system (e.g. heart) or part of a body system (e.g. motor system in the legs). The subject is usually a volunteer (often a fellow student at a different stage in the course) and will not have any medical problems (no abnormal physical signs). The question that the examiner asks is straight-forward ('Please show me how you would examine the respiratory system') and the criteria for marking are based on the steps required of the standard examination ('did the candidate percuss the chest in an adequate manner?').

You can prepare for this basic competency examination by the following:

1. List the body systems and any subdivisions (e.g. heart, peripheral vascular system).
2. Work through this list, focussing on one system at a time (e.g. respiratory system).
3. Acquire competence in the examination by **practising** it, not by reading about it or watching a video.
4. Use books and videos to remind you of the steps.
5. Practise the skill on fellow students/clinical partners, patients (who do not have abnormal physical signs in that system).
6. Use the 'responses and commentaries' in the book to judge your performance.
7. Speed up acquisition of the skill by 'talking through the steps' of the examination (e.g. 'now I assess the character of the pulse at the carotid artery') at the same time as practising it (unless instructed, you will not do this in the OSCE).
8. Practise the skill with a clinical partner, who can observe your examination and grade your performance according to the core skills and commentaries. You can then do the same for them (and learn by observation of their technique).

ADVANCED LEVEL

The stations in the OSCE may be longer (10–15 min) and may involve examining patients with physical signs, interpreting these and suggesting investigations or a management plan. Sometimes examination of a patient (e.g. heart) might be coupled with listening to an audiotape (or CAL programme) of a physical sign (e.g. *If you had heard this when you were listening to the patient, how would you interpret it?*).

The steps involved in preparation for an advanced level OSCE are very similar to those outlined for the basic exam. You must have consolidated the basic examination technique before you can use it to elicit physical signs. The analogy is with riding a bike; you first have to master the skill of riding then use it to take you to where you want to go.

The major difference between basic and advanced skills is the competence to determine whether a physical sign is present or absent. So how do you acquire this confidence? The glib answer is by gaining as much experience as possible. More useful, is to focus on what is likely to appear in the OSCE.

Using neurology as the example, consider what physical conditions are:

- Stable, so the signs do not change
- In plentiful supply, so that similar patients can be used to examine all students.

It follows that conditions like stroke and peripheral neuropathy (diabetes) are the ones that you are most likely to encounter in the exam. Therefore, you prepare for the OSCE (once you are happy with your basic neurological examination) by:

- Seeking out such patients and examining them (e.g. stroke rehabilitation ward, out-patient clinic for diabetes).

You should also seek opportunities to exam any patient with neurological signs. It is only possible to make judgement on the presence of 'increased tone' if you have examined:

1. Lots of people with normal tone.
2. Some people with high tone in the arms or legs.

DEMONSTRATION OF COMPETENCE IN THE EXAM

At both the basic and advanced stages, competence is judged by the examiner using a number of criteria:

- Did you go through all the steps listed in the marking schedule?
- Was the technique you used for the steps (e.g. palpation) adequate?
- Did you look as though you had performed the exam before? This is quite easy to judge by whether your examination flowed from one step to another or you had to keep stopping and thinking.
- Was the overall examination of high standard? (did you 'put it all together').
- At the advanced level, the examiner will also assess whether you can interpret what you have found and use appropriate language (without lots of qualifiers such as *There might possibly be a slight hint of a murmer, but I am not sure!*).

You can improve your performance by practising with colleagues and marking each other. Even better is to persuade a house officer or someone senior to watch you and give a judgement on your competence and how you can improve it. The more senior the member of staff, the more it will simulate the exam and help to polish your performance for the big day.

USING THIS SECTION OF THE BOOK

As with the other sections, we have tried to include most of the common scenarios you will face. In this chapter, the station has a description of the basic examination technique. If you are unsure of anything, you must go to one of the standard clinical examination textbooks or videos for more detail.

Some stations are set at an advanced level by asking you to indicate what physical signs you might expect with a particular diagnosis or what diagnosis you might reach given a set of physical signs. We have also included 'station extensions' to show how real patients or data can be used to increase the complexity.

You will get the most out of the section by running through the stations and either:

- writing down what you would do if asked *'Please show me how you would examine this patient's shoulder'*.
  or (preferably)
- going through the station with a partner watching you examine a patient (with or without a shoulder problem).

| EXAMINATION 1 | **Measure the blood pressure** |

Level:	*
Setting:	Volunteer patient (student) or a mannequin arm. Available will be sphygmomanometer and cuffs of various sizes
Time:	5 min

TASK

E – *Please take this person's blood pressure and tell me the reading.*

RESPONSE

Measuring the blood pressure is a basic skill that many people do badly, particularly when checked against standard criteria (see core skill box).

> **Core skill: Measurement of blood pressure**
>
> The key steps (in order) are:
>
> 1. Check that the sphygmomanometer is working and set to zero.
> 2. Choose an appropriate cuff size.
> 3. Wrap the cuff neatly around the arm with the bladder over the brachial artery.
> 4. Support the arm at the level of the heart.
> 5. Inflate the cuff whilst palpating the radial or brachial artery and determine the systolic pressure by palpation.
> 6. Inflate the cuff back to 20–30 mmHg over the systolic pressure and let the pressure out slowly.
> 7. Record the systolic and diastolic pressure to the nearest 2 mmHg.
> 8. State that you would recheck the blood pressure with the person standing.

In detail, the steps are:

1. Make sure you have the correct size of cuff – obese patients need large cuffs, children small. If you take the blood pressure in an obese patient with a standard cuff, you will get a falsely high reading as the cuff has to exert a greater pressure to compress the artery.
2. Inflate the cuff whilst palpating the radial or brachial artery to obtain the systolic pressure *by palpation*. Inflate 20–30 mmHg above where you cannot feel pulsation. Let the pressure out slowly until you feel the pulse return.

3. Use either the bell or diaphragm to obtain the blood pressure by auscultation. A critical point is to inflate the cuff back to 20–30 mmHg over the systolic pressure by palpation. Let the pressure out slowly (2 mmHg/s).
4. The point at which you hear the first Korotkof sound is the systolic pressure. Record this to the nearest *2 mmHg*.
5. Continue to deflate. The point at which the sounds *disappear* (Korotkof Vth sound) is the diastolic pressure. Again record to nearest 2 mmHg. In some normal people, the sounds may not disappear, then use Korotkof IVth sound (muffling) and record that you have done this.
6. State that you would go on to measure the blood pressure with the patient standing to check for a postural drop.
7. If there is a drop of 20 mmHg systolic pressure that is still present (sustained) at 2 minutes then the patient has postural hypotension.

Extension to station (Level: **)

The station can incorporate a mannequin arm that allows the examiner to set (and reset) the blood pressure so that they can judge whether you are accurate in your measurement.

EXAMINATION 2 | # Heart examination

Level:	*
Setting:	Volunteer patient (student)
Time:	5 min

TASK

E – *Please examine the patient's heart excluding the blood pressure.*

RESPONSE

The steps in the examination of the heart are given in the core skill box.

Core skill: Examination of the heart

In your basic heart examination, you should:

1. Position the patient correctly and expose the chest at the right time.

2. Inspect and comment on the presence or absence of abnormality (e.g. patient not breathless at rest).

3. Examine the hands for abnormalities (e.g. clubbing, splinter haemorrhages).

4. Feel and comment on the pulse (radial and carotid) – rate, rhythm, character.

5. Demonstrate the jugular venous pulse (by changing position of patient).

6. Palpate the chest for apex beat and thrills.

7. Use the bell of your stethoscope to listen over the heart in the four areas.

8. Demonstrate the additional manoeuvres to bring out aortic incompetence (using the diaphragm) and mitral stenosis (using the bell).

9. Examine for dependent oedema.

Position

The patient should usually be positioned with the trunk at 45°. There is nothing magical about this – it is simply the angle at which the jugular venous pressure should just be visible in the root of the neck (1–2 cm above the manubrio-sternal joint). Overriding anything is the comfort of the patient – if they are only able to sit up without distress then you examine them in this position.

The patient is asked to remove their top clothing to expose the chest. In female patients, it is better to leave her bra on until you need to listen to the heart. **Always put the dignity of the patient top of your considerations**.

Inspection

The best place to observe the patient is the foot of the bed. Ask yourself (and comment on) whether the patient looks blue (cyanosed). Central cyanosis is seen around the lips and tongue. Is the patient tachypnoeic at rest – count the respirations, are they above 20?

Look at the hands
Is the patient clubbed? Are the hands cold (vasoconstriction, poor perfusion) or warm (vasodilatation). Are the nail beds blue – peripheral cyanosis.

Palpation
Feel the radial pulse. Is it present? Feel for the opposite side, is it equal? What is the rhythm – regular or irregular? If irregular, how does it vary? If no pattern – most likely it is atrial fibrillation, but you should state that you would confirm this with an ECG. What is the rate? Count over 15–20 seconds and average over a minute. Remember: tachycardia is > 100 beats per min, bradycardia is < 60 beats per min.

The character of the pulse is best assessed at the carotid artery. There are two other classical methods:

1. Place your thumb over the brachial artery in the antecubital fossa. Plateau (slow rising pulse – aortic stenosis) pulse.
2. Lift the patient's arm above the patient's head. Place your palm across the wrist – you will feel the radial artery knocking on your hand. Collapsing pulse (aortic incompetence).

Observe around the head
You should look for central cyanosis (tongue) and anaemia (very difficult sign – conjunctiva).

Jugular venous pressure
Identify pulsation by looking at a tangent across the side of the neck. Ask the patient to look away from you and observe pulsation beneath the sternomastoid. You are not looking for the external, but the internal vein. If you see pulsation, *the next question is 'is it venous'?*

- You cannot palpate venous pulsation
- You can 'obliterate it' by pressing over the root of the neck
- If you press over the abdomen (right hypochondrium) the pressure rises (abomino-jugular reflex [hepato-jugular])
- Venous pulsation has a double impulse (A and V waves).

If you are convinced that pulsation is venous – measure its vertical height from the manubrio-sternal joint. You can make venous pulsation visible in almost anybody by getting them to lie flatter than 45°.

Apex beat and thrills

Over the praecordium you should try to identify the apex beat (difficult/impossible in a lot of people). If you find it – ask yourself where it is in relation to the clavicle and rib space, it should be in the mid-clavicular line, 5th intercostal space. Ask yourself what is the character of the apex beat: is it 'tapping' on your hand (loud 1st heart sound – mitral stenosis) or is it 'heaving' (left ventricular hypertrophy)?

Feel for 'thrills' (turbulent blood flow – indicating the presence of a murmur) by placing either the heel of your hand or all your fingers over:

- the apex – mitral area
- left sternal edge, 4th interspace – tricuspid area
- left sternal edge, 2nd interspace – pulmonary area
- right sternal edge, 2nd interspace – aortic area

Using the bell of your stethoscope listen over the heart in the four areas listed.

Ask yourself:

1. Are there any murmurs? If so are they in systole or diastole? Do they occupy all of systole (pansystolic – cannot hear 2nd heart sound clearly) or are they in the middle (midsystolic – can hear the 2nd heart sound)? You can time a murmur by palpating over the carotid artery (pulse = systole) – this is quite difficult. Where does the murmur radiate to (neck, axilla)?
2. What are the heart sounds like – are they soft or loud? Is the second heart sound split (normal on inspiration)?
3. Are there any added sounds – 3rd heart sound (just after 2nd heart sound) or 4th heart sound (just before 1st heart sound)?
4. Is there a pericardial rub (scratching sound in systole and diastole)?

There are two additional manoeuvres:

1. Turn the patient slightly over onto their left side. Ask the patient to 'breath in, breath out, hold it there'. Listen with the bell for the low pitched rumbling mid-diastolic murmur of mitral stenosis (with a loud 1st heart sound).
2. Sit the patient forward, ask them to again take a deep breath in, breath out and hold it. Listen with the diaphragm over the aortic area and the left sternal edge for the high pitched blowing early diastolic murmur of aortic incompetence.

Remember: Most of the sounds from the heart are low pitched and these are best picked up using the bell of the stethoscope. This is particularly true of mitral stenosis. The exception is the high pitched murmur of aortic incompetence – listen with a diaphragm.

Examine for dependent oedema

Usually this is over the ankles/feet. With firm consistent pressure, press over the anterior tibial border for 10 seconds. If oedema is present you will see 'pitting' – an indentation where your finger has been. Remember, if a patient has been in bed for a long time then the oedema may be over the sacrum – check here.

Table 4.1 Physical signs of heart failure

Valve	Murmur	Other signs
Aortic	Stenosis: Mid-systolic, best heard aortic area	Plateau pulse, narrow pulse pressure, soft second heart sound, left ventricular hypertrophy
	Incompetence: Early diastolic, blowing, high pitched (diaphragm). Best heard left sternal edge	Collapsing pulse, pulsation in nail bed. Displaced apex beat
Mitral	Stenosis: Mid-diastolic, rumbling, best heard apex Incompetence: Pan-systolic, best heard apex, but wide radiation. Goes up to 2nd heart sound	Tapping apex, loud first heart sound, opening snap (pliant valve)
Tricuspid	Stenosis: Very rare – 'small print' Incompetence: Pan-systolic, best heard left sternal edge, 4th or 5th interspace. Murmur varies with respiration	Giant V waves, pulsatile liver
Pulmonary	Stenosis: Rare. Mid-systolic murmur, 2nd left interspace Incompetence: Very rare – 'small print'	Soft second heart sound
Other abnormalities		
Ventricular septal defect	Pan-systolic murmur, loud	Cyanosis (pulmonary hypertension), clubbing
Atrial septal defect		Wide fixed splitting of 2nd heart sound

SUGGESTIONS FOR FURTHER PRACTICE

As with the respiratory examination, acutely ill patients often have cardiovascular signs – heart failure, raised JVP and murmurs (commonest is pansystolic – mitral or tricuspid incompetence).

Specialist cardiac out-patient clinics will have patients with physical signs that you often do not see (or hear) elsewhere – murmurs of aortic valve disease and mitral stenosis. Many units run 'Heart failure' clinics – these offer good experience as the patients are relatively stable (unlike in hospital).

Extensions to station (Levels: **/***)

There are several ways that you may encounter a more advanced station:

- Using patients with stable physical signs. Alternatively, a patient with a normal cardiovascular system can be linked to a recording of valvular disease. The physical signs are summarised in Table 4.1.
- Interpretation of ECGs (and other data) – see Data 2: Chest radiograph and Procedure 1: Record an ECG.

EXAMINATION 3	Peripheral vascular examination
Level:	***
Setting:	A patient with intermittent claudication
Time:	5–10 min

TASK

E – *This patient is complaining of pain in his legs when he walks about 100 yards. I want you to examine his peripheral vascular system and comment on your findings as you go along.*

RESPONSE

A key element in this station is *talking the examiner through your examination and findings*. The examiner may become irritated if they keep having to remind you to do this, particularly as the patient does have some physical signs and to get the marks, you have to say what these are.

Expose the whole of the lower limbs from the groin down to the feet. If not, you may miss an operation scar (e.g. femoro-popliteal bypass) or nail changes due to ischaemia.

Inspection

Comment on:

- Obvious signs of (pre) gangrene – blackness, missing toes, nail infection.
- Ulceration – if present, you need to describe the ulcer (size, shape, bed, edge, slough, surrounding skin) and consider whether it is likely to be venous (varicose veins, varicose eczema, usually painless) or arterial ('punched out', painful).
- Skin changes – staining due to previous ulceration, varicose eczema), loss of hair on extremities, pallor.
- Varicose veins – best seen with person standing. At the front and medial aspect, you may observe tortuous, dilated branches of the long saphenous vein from below the femoral vein in the groin to the medial side of the lower leg. At the back, you may see varicosities of the short saphenous veins from the popliteal fossa to the posterior calf and lateral malleolus. Comment on any inflammation or superficial phlebitis.
- Scars from operations – groin, medial aspect of thigh.

> **Core skill: Examination of the peripheral vascular system**
>
> 1. Expose the whole of the lower limbs.
>
> 2. Inspection:
>   - Signs of (pre) gangrene
>   - Any ulceration – describe
>   - Skin changes – varicose eczema, loss of hair, pallor
>   - Varicose veins – best seen with person standing
>   - Scars from operations.
>
> 3. Palpation:
>   - Peripheral pulses (femoral, popliteal, posterior tibial, dorsalis pedis)
>   - Difference in skin temperature
>   - Look for reduced capillary return
>   - Palpate any varicosities.
>
> 4. Auscultation – femoral artery and aorta.

Palpation

Examine the peripheral pulses:

- Femoral – over inguinal ligament
- Popliteal – with the knee flexed and foot resting on the bed, wrap your hands around the knee, placing both sets of fingers in the popliteal space (this is a difficult technique to master)
- Posterior tibial – behind the medial malleolus
- Dorsalis pedis – over dorsum of the foot. Slide your fingers up from the 1st metatarsal space.

With each pulse, comment on how strong it is – particularly in comparison with the pulse in the opposite leg. You should also palpate the radial and femoral pulse together for 'femoral delay' – coarctation.

Comment on any difference in skin temperature. Use the back of your hand and compare the two legs starting at the feet and moving up the limb (if normal and no difference at the feet, then little point in proceeding).

Look for reduced capillary return by compressing a nail bed and estimate how long the normal red colour takes to return. If it is slow, you can perform Buerger's test in which you elevate the leg to 45° (pallor develops rapidly with a poor arterial supply) and then place the legs dependent at 90° over the edge of the couch (cyanosis occurs).

If the patient has got varicose veins, you should palpate these to see if there is any hardness or tenderness suggesting thrombophlebitis.

Auscultation

Listen over the femoral artery and aorta (abdomen) for bruits.

SUGGESTIONS FOR FURTHER PRACTICE

The best place to see patients with peripheral vascular disease is in a vascular surgical clinic. However, this does not mean that such patients would be confined to surgical OSCEs, as intermittent claudication is very common in medical practice.

Extension to station (Level: ***)

This station could be changed in a number of ways. A volunteer with no abnormalities could be used to determine whether you can perform the basic examination. This could be linked to a photograph of a patient with gangrene, diabetic foot problems or an arteriogram.

EXAMINATION 4	**Respiratory examination 1**
Level:	*
Setting:	**Volunteer patient (student) on a couch**
Time:	5 mln

TASK

E – *Please show me how you would examine the respiratory system.*

RESPONSE

> ### Core skill: Examination of the respiratory system
>
> The key steps are:
>
> 1. Adequate general inspection with appropriate comments on specific aspects (e.g. tachypnoea).
>
> 2. Examination of the hands for clubbing, peripheral cyanosis, peripheral vasodilatation, and 'flap' (asterixis).
>
> 3. Examination of the head and neck for central cyanosis and lymphadenopathy.
>
> 4. Palpation including tracheal deviation, apex beat and chest expansion (front and back).
>
> 5. Percussion over chest wall including apices and lateral chest wall.
>
> 6. Tactile vocal fremitus.
>
> 7. Auscultation – comment on breath sounds and added sounds.
>
> 8. Vocal resonance.

General inspection

Always start this when you are talking to the patient – look for (*and comment to the examiner*) breathlessness (tachypnoea), cyanosis, breathing through pursed lips, 'wet' cough etc. At the end of the bed you should look for:

● Respiratory rate (tachypnoea > 20/min)
● Use of accessory muscles
● Rib cage deformity
● Equality of movement of chest wall on both sides.

HANDS

Look for clubbing (loss of angle, nail bed fluctuation, increased curvature both planes). Be very careful about using the phrase *'early clubbing'*; because this has diagnostic implications, the examiner will wake up and want to ask questions! Are there signs of carbon dioxide retention (warm peripheries, dilated veins, bounding pulse)?

Examine for a *'flap'* (*asterixis*), which is a coarse, irregular jerking of the hands at the wrists):

- Ask the patient to put their hands outstretched
- Ask them to cock up their wrists (extension)
- Observe for 30 seconds.

Head and neck

Look for central cyanosis (tongue) and use of accessory muscles. Examine for lymph nodes in the cervical chain, supra and infraclavicular fossae and axillae.

Chest

It is easier to examine the front of the chest completely, then move on to the back. Compare each side as you move through the examination.

Palpation

1. Tracheal deviation: (*A difficult sign – i.e. not of great use and examiners have different techniques and opinions.*) Place your index and middle finger either side of the trachea in the suprasternal notch. There should be equal spacing. Deviation of the trachea occurs with *upper* lobe collapse.
2. Chest expansion (front and back): Place your hands on the person's chest with your fingers spread outwards and your palms close to the midline. Your thumbs should be pointing towards the head of the patient. Your fingers should be firmly applied and your thumbs 'floating'. Observe the movement with normal breathing and then ask the person to take a deep breath in. Observe any differences between the two sides. Normal chest expansion is at least 5 cm (you can measure it).

Percussion
You should percuss all down the chest on both sides. At the front there will be areas of dullness due to the liver on the right and the heart on the left. Remember to percuss for the apices of the lungs over the clavicles.

Tactile vocal fremitus
(This is the equivalent of vocal resonance and is not as good.) Over the chest wall in the upper, mid and lower zones, place the side of your hand (medial border) firmly against the chest. Ask the patient to say '99' and compare the two sides.

Auscultation

Use either the bell or the diaphragm. Listen over the upper, mid and lower zones comparing sides. The sounds should be 'vesicular'.

Added sounds can be:

1. Wheezes (rhonchi) – musical quality
2. Crackles (crepitations).

The vesicular breath sounds may be diminished because the lung is not aerated or there is something in the way of their conduction to the stethoscope (e.g. pleural fluid). If the lung is consolidated then you may hear *bronchial breathing*.

Vocal resonance

Whilst listening to the upper, mid and lower zones ask the patient to say '99'. Compare the two sides. Are they equal? Is one side soft or loud?

You need to repeat the steps (see Core skill box) on the back of the chest.

EXAMINATION SKILLS

EXAMINATION SKILLS

EXAMINATION 5 — Respiratory examination 2

Level:	**
Setting:	A patient with respiratory signs
Time:	10 min

TASK

E – *This patient is complaining of breathlessness. Please examine their respiratory system and tell me what your diagnosis is.*

Later, the examiner asks you:

E – *What signs might you have found in this patient if they had:*

a. Pleural effusion
b. Fibrosis alveolitis
c. Chronic bronchitis and emphysema
d. Lobar consolidation.

RESPONSE

In an OSCE, all candidates should be assessed in a standard way. However, inclusion of patients introduces some variability into a station, which needs to be minimised. A station designed to include a patient with 'any respiratory disease' is too vague and would lead to some students seeing 'easy' things and some being assessed on patients with rare problems or 'tricky' signs. So the organisers have to use common problems that have stable, **definite**, physical signs.

In the list for this station, although knowledge about the signs of consolidation, or of a pneumothorax may come up in a data interpretation station (e.g. interpret this chest radiograph), it would be impossible in a large scale OSCE to find enough patients with these problems.

> **Core skill: Detection and interpretation of respiratory signs**
>
> The skills are the same as in Examination 4 with the addition of:
>
> 1. Elicit the physical signs.
>
> 2. Interpret these correctly.
>
> 3. Know the physical signs associated with respiratory disease, shown in Table 4.2.

In the list of options given by the examiner, the most likely problem you will

Table 4.2 Physical signs found in common chest problems

Disease	Chest movement	Percussion note	Breath sounds	Added sounds	Vocal resonance	Other signs/notes
Pleural effusion	May be reduced if massive effusion	Stony Dull	Reduced	None	Reduced	May be mediastinal shift (apex beat) if massive
Consolidation	No change	Dull	Bronchial Breathing	None or some localised crackles	Increased ('whispering pectoriloquy')	Bronchial breathing is often transient. May be tachypnoeic
Pneumothorax	May be reduced	Increased resonance	Reduced, vesicular (Silent – if tension)	None	Reduced	Tracheal deviation if tension. Also cyanosis
Lobar collapse	No change	Slight reduction	Slight reduced, vesicular	None or few crackles	Slight reduction	Characterised by 'slight reduction in everthing'. Better diagnosed by radiograph
Asthma	Reduced	No change or slight increase in resonance	Reduced, vesicular (Silent – if severe)	Widespread expiratory wheezes	No change	
Chronic bronchitis and emphysema	Reduced	Increase in resonance	Reduced, vesicular	Widespread expiratory wheezes	No change	Evidence of congestive cardiac failure
Pulmonary fibrosis (fibrosing alveolitis)	No change	No change	Vesicular	Fine, late inspiratory crackles	No change	Clubbed, particularly in cryptogenic fibrosing alveolitis

encounter in an OSCE is chronic airflow obstruction (e.g. chronic asthma or chronic bronchitis and emphysema), followed by pulmonary fibrosis.

SUGGESTIONS FOR FURTHER PRACTICE

Respiratory signs are common in patients admitted as acute medical emergencies. In these patients the signs you are most likely to encounter are wheezes and crackles. If a patient has a pleural effusion, make sure that you are confident that you can elicit the signs. Bronchial breathing is usually transient. So, in an OSCE, the best way of introducing this physical sign is through a recording. (There are very good CAL packages available on cardiac and respiratory signs – have you seen whether your library/skills centre has a programme?)

Extension to station (Level: ***)

The station can be extended by the addition of data or images. These could be:

- Blood gases – see Data 6: Deliberate self-harm and Procedure 15: Arterial blood sampling.
- Spirometry. The patterns you must be able to recognise are:
  - Obstructive (reduced FEV_1/FVC ratio)
  - Restrictive (Both FEV_1 and FVC reduced, ratio normal, > 70%).
- Peak expiratory flow rate – particularly the diurnal variation of asthma.
- Radiographs (see Fig. 4.1). The station may be extended thus:

TASK

E – *Describe the abnormalities you see on this radiograph. What physical signs might you expect the patient to have?*

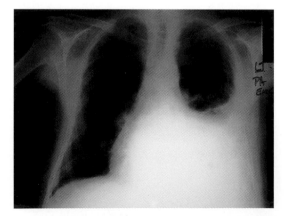

Figure 4.1

RESPONSE

The patient has a left pleural effusion. The costophrenic angle is obliterated with a concave shadow tracking up the pleural margin. You would expect the physical signs indicated in Table 4.2. The key skill of interpretation of chest radiographs is discussed in Data 2: Chest radiograph.

EXAMINATION SKILLS

EXAMINATION 6 # Examine the abdomen

Level:	*/**
Setting:	Volunteer patient (student) laid on a couch
Time:	5 min

TASK

E – *Please show me how you would examine the patient's abdomen other than the groin/pubis area? I want you to describe what you are doing/looking for as you go along.*

RESPONSE

Core skill: Abdominal examination

1. Inspection:
   - General
   - Hands
   - Head and neck
   - Abdomen.

2. Position of patient.

3. Palpation:
   - General
   - Liver
   - Spleen
   - Kidneys.

4. Percussion:
   - Shifting dullness
   - Liver
   - Bladder.

5. Auscultation.

6. Hernia orifices.

7. Genitalia.

8. Rectal examination.

A sample interaction between the student and examiner may go along the following lines:

S – *The first thing I will do is to make sure the patient is comfortable and lying flat with one pillow for support – (to patient – 'Are you alright like that Mr Johnson?'). I am now starting with the hands looking for clubbing, palmar erythema (liver disease), and a Dupuytren's contracture (cirrhosis).*
(To patient – 'Could you put your hands out like this and cock your wrists up, now just hold it like that'.) I am now looking for a flap.

E – *Do you get a flap in any other condition?*

S – *You may see it with respiratory failure as a sign of carbon dioxide retention.*

E – *Good.*

S – *I am now moving to the head and neck (to patient – 'Can you look up to the ceiling for me?'). I look for jaundice in the sclera.*

E – *What level of bilirubin can you detect as jaundice?*

S – *When it is at least four times the upper limit of normal range.*

E – *A bit too much, usually twice – so over 36 µmol/L.*

S – *I am also looking for anaemia and I will examine for lymphadenopathy.*

S – *(To patient – 'Can you open your mouth for me, Mr Johnson?') I am looking for ulcers as these can be a sign of Crohn's disease.*
(To patient – 'May I take your shirt off?')
I am now examining the upper body for gynaecomastia and spider naevi.

E – *What is the significance of these?*

S – *Well, in a man, gynaecomastia is seen in cirrhosis in which you get high circulating oestrogen levels because the liver does not break down the hormone. Similarly, with spider naevi, except you can have up to 5 in a woman who is not pregnant.*

S – *(To patient) 'May I just pull this blanket down to feel your stomach?'*
The first thing I do is to see whether the abdomen is distended at all.

E – *What if it was?*

S – *Well, I remember that general swelling can be due to 'fs' – fluid, flatus, fat, faeces and a fetus in woman.*

E – *What else are you looking for?*

S – *Is the abdomen moving with respiration – because if not then patient could have a rigid abdomen, which is a sign of peritonitis. I am also looking to see if there are any masses visible.*

At this point, the examiner may let you get on with it, as they are satisfied that you are not simply following steps, but have knowledge of why you are looking for certain signs. In the remainder of your examination, you should go on to:

Palpation

You must do this in a systematic manner. Your arm should be parallel to the skin surface. This means that you will have to sit or kneel in many cases. You should ask the patient if there is any tenderness – so that you can take this into account. With the palmar aspect of all your fingers of your *right* hand, you should *superficially* palpate each of the regions in turn (see Fig. 4.2). You should

EXAMINATION SKILLS

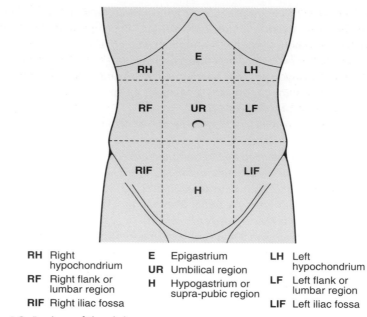

RH Right hypochondrium	**E** Epigastrium	**LH** Left hypochondrium
RF Right flank or lumbar region	**UR** Umbilical region	**LF** Left flank or lumbar region
RIF Right iliac fossa	**H** Hypogastrium or supra-pubic region	**LIF** Left iliac fossa

Figure 4.2 Regions of the abdomen

be looking at the patient's face for any signs of tenderness/pain. Ask yourself whether:

- The abdomen feels soft – is there any local guarding?
- Are there any masses? – If so, you will have to describe them – position, shape, size, surface, fixed, movement with respiration, tenderness, pulsation (transmitted or direct).
- You should repeat the palpation but going deeper.

Specific palpation

There are a number of organs that you should specifically examine for:

1. *Liver:* The liver enlarges down the abdomen. Ask the patient to take some deep breaths. As they breathe in, the liver is displaced down and you should move your fingers up towards the right hypochondrium. If you feel an edge, then you have to describe it as with an abdominal mass. Is the edge smooth or irregular, is it tender, are there any nodules over its surface? You must quantify any enlargement by approximate measurement in centimetres (not finger breadths) from the costal margin.
2. *Spleen:* The spleen enlarges towards the right iliac fossa. Using the same technique as with the liver, move your hand up the abdomen with each breath towards the left hypochondrium. There are two techniques which can help you palpate a spleen. One is to ask the patient to draw up their knees to relax their abdominal musculature. The other is to lie the patient on their right side facing you with their knees drawn up. This allows the spleen to fall away from the ribs. Palpation is then by the usual technique.

3. *Kidneys:* The kidneys are palpated by balotting them bimanually. What this means is that your watching/detecting hand (right) palpates in the renal areas (flanks) and your other hand (left) is underneath the patient in the renal angle (between the 12th rib and the spine). As the patient breathes in and out, the lower hand pushes the kidney towards the watching hand (balots). In most people the kidneys are not palpable. You may feel them in very thin people. The right kidney is lower than the left. The kidneys move on respiration and percussion may be resonant over them because of the overlying bowel.

Percussion

- You should percuss over the liver area to detect any enlargement on the liver that you can then confirm by palpation. The upper border should be around the 4th intercostal space and the lower border is at the costal margin.
- You should percuss suprapubically listening for dullness suggestive of bladder distension. It is often easier to detect this way than by palpation.
- The other main use of percussion is testing for *shifting dullness* in ascites. If a patient has a distended abdomen (see above) you need to consider whether this is due to ascites. If the abdomen is not distended, there is little point in carrying out this manoeuvre.
  1. First, percuss from the umbilicus laterally (with your fingers pointing towards the head) and ascertain that the percussion note is resonant at the umbilicus (gas at the apex) and dull in the flanks (fluid – dependent). If this is not the case, then the patient does not have ascites.
  2. Secondly, ask the patient to roll over towards you (on their right side), whilst keeping your hand over the left flank where it was dull. Wait for approx 30 s then percuss again. The fluid should drain towards you, and the gas towards the left flank. Percuss again over your fingers – the note should now be resonant
  3. Thirdly, roll the patient over to their left side, wait and percuss. The note over the left flank should be dull again. In the right flank it should be resonant.

Auscultation

At the end of the examination, you should auscultate close to the umbilicus for bowel sounds (increased, reduced, absent). You should also listen for bruits – aorta. A complete abdominal examination would also include examination of the hernia orifices, genital (see Examination 8) and rectal examination (see Examination 7).

SUGGESTION FOR FURTHER PRACTICE

Apart from gastrointestinal and liver clinics, other specialities in which you will encounter patients with abdominal signs include:

- Haematology clinics – many patients with hepatosplenomegaly, and the best place to convince yourself of what an enlarged spleen feels like.

- Renal units – easily palpable kidneys are rare in general medicine. In an exam, the most likely cause of enlarged kidneys would be polycystic disease.
- Oncology units – patients with gastrointestinal tumours and hepatic metastases.

Extensions to stations (Levels: **/***)

The easiest way to extend the station would be to include:

- A patient with chronic liver disease – here the stigmata are likely to be predominantly **away** from the abdomen.
- A patient with hepatomegaly.
- Other organomegaly would be unusual for an OSCE that involved a large number of students – it would be difficult to obtain patients with similar signs.

EXAMINATION 7	**Rectal examination**
Level:	*/**
Setting:	A pelvic mannequin (male or female)
Time:	5 min

TASK

E – *Please perform a rectal examination on this mannequin. Please talk to me as if I am the patient.*

RESPONSE

A hard part of this station is to pretend that you are talking to a real patient. The examiner will also find it a contrived thing to do. The educational reason for including it is that it encourages you to find the simple words that are necessary to explain a procedure to a patient. When learning, most students tend not to be very conformable about telling patients what to do. They become quiet and mumble. They also use a lot of technical terms that patients cannot necessarily understand. The more you practice the phrases (e.g. *I would now like to examine your back passage*) the more it becomes a habit that transfers into clinical practice. The other reason for you doing so in this station is that there will be marks for it!

> **Core skill: Rectal examination**
>
> 1. Seek a chaperone (if appropriate).
> 2. Obtain consent.
> 3. Give clear instructions to the mannequin during the examination (or examiner).
> 4. Inspect the anus and surrounding area.
> 5. Prepare the gloved finger with lubricant.
> 6. Insert the finger through the rectum using a posterior approach.
> 7. Rotate the hand to examine the prostate and rectal wall.
> 8. Wipe the anus with the gauze at the end of the examination.

You must be able to perform a rectal examination, but it is a very difficult technique to obtain adequate practice given the sensitivities involved. Using mannequins is an adequate substitute whilst acquiring and consolidating the basic technique. Regardless of the gender of the patient, it is good practice to have a nurse with you when performing a rectal examination.

EXAMINATION SKILLS

The steps involved are:

1. Inform the patient what you want to do and why it is necessary: *I need to examine the back passage using my finger to see whether there are any problems there. Is that alright?*
2. Get the patient in the correct position. The person should be asked to turn onto their left hand side, with their knees drawn up towards the chest. The chaperone should be on the left hand side of the bed so that they can reassure the patient.
3. Inspect the anus and surrounding skin. For example, look for skin tags, ulcers, prolapsed piles, fissures. If the patient has a fissure, rectal examination may be too painful.
4. Apply lubricant to the gloved index finger of your right hand.
5. Tell the patient that they may feel some pressure and discomfort. They should take *'easy breaths'*.
6. Insert your finger. From the back of the patient run your finger along the midline to the anus. Exert pressure on the anus towards the back and gently push your finger into the rectum.
7. Examine the rectum in a systematic manner. You will have to sweep your finger around the rectum by rotating your hand clockwise and anticlockwise.
8. Ask yourself the following questions:
   a. is the rectum loaded with faeces – it should usually be empty
   b. are the faeces hard or soft – alters treatment for constipation
   c. is there any intrinsic lesion of the rectum – hard edge of a carcinoma
   d. does the prostate feel normal – is it enlarged, is it irregular, is there any nodule
   e. is the midline groove lost?
9. Remove your finger and examine the glove:
   a. is there any blood, mucus
   b. are the faeces black – malaena or iron therapy.
10. Wipe the anus with gauze, dispose of the glove.

SUGGESTIONS FOR FURTHER PRACTICE

Have you been to the skills laboratory outside any scheduled activity and used the mannequins? They will be the same (or very similar) to those used in the exam. In relation to patients, the best units in which you are likely to have opportunities to practice rectal examinations are in urology and gastroenterology.

Extension to station (Level: **)

The station could be extended by using one of the mannequins that offers examples of different prostate abnormalities (benign enlargement through to local maligant invasion) – has your skills laboratory got such a model? Prostatic enlargement could be coupled with a radiograph showing metastatic disease (sclerosing), or a raised prostatic specific antigen.

EXAMINATION 8	**Male genital examination**
Level:	*
Setting:	Examination on a male pelvic mannequin
Time:	5 min

TASK

E – *Please show me how you would examine the genitalia.*

RESPONSE

This station is very common in OSCEs looking at competency in basic skills (like rectal examination). It was rarely examined before the advent of good quality teaching mannequins and many students never acquired the skill. Sometimes the examiner may ask you to 'talk to the model as if it was a real patient'. This is very difficult, but the major reason for including it in the marking criteria is to signal that the more you practise what to say, the easier it will become with patients. You should wear gloves for the examination.

Core skill: Examination of the male genitalia

1. If asked – talk to the model or examiner.

2. Inspection – ulcers/lesions around the penis and scrotum. Mucosal ulceration and urethral discharge

3. Note whether the left testis is slightly lower. Palpate each testis and vas deferens, and comment on its presence, shape, size, consistency and any associated masses.

4. Trans-illuminate any masses.

Inspection

Comment on any ulcers/lesions around the penis and scrotum. You should look for mucosal ulceration around the glans penis (gently retract the foreskin) and urethral discharge. (You should state that any discharge would be sent for microscopic examination and culture).

Look at the scrotum. Usually the left testis hangs slightly lower than the right. Palpate each testis, epididymus and vas deferens gently using the finger and thumb of your hand. The testes should be equal in size, smooth and firm. An absent testis may be due to failure of descent, surgical removal (tumour, torsion)

or retraction. You should feel for an undescended testis in the inguinal canal. Small testes suggests endocrine disease (hypogonadism).

If you feel a mass in the scrotum:

- Can you get above it (if not – consider hernia).
- If it is confined to the scrotum
  - Is it separate or part of the testis
  - Can you trans-illuminate it.

A solid testicular mass is likely to be a tumour (e.g. seminoma, teratoma). A hydrocoele is cystic mass with the testis within it. You should also consider varicocoele, which will feel like a mass of soft cords posterior to the testes, extending up the epididymus.

SUGGESTIONS FOR FURTHER PRACTICE

During your studies, you need to plan when you are going to go to the skills laboratory and practise various skills on the mannequins. It may be that the laboratory allows you to 'drop in' at any time or you may need to book time.

EXAMINATION SKILLS

EXAMINATION 9 — Examine higher cortical function

Level:	***
Setting:	Examine a patient with a stroke
Time:	10 min

TASK

E – *Mr Hussain has had a stroke. It has caused him some problems. I would like you to show me how you would assess his higher cortical function.*

RESPONSE

This is a difficult station. You have to consider what higher functions you can easily test 'at the bedside' and where they might be localised. You could draw on your experience of performing mental state examination in psychiatry. A basic checklist is shown in the box:

Core skill: Examination of higher cognitive function

1. Language – dysphasia, dyslexia, dysgraphia.

2. Ten-point mental test score, which includes tests of orientation.

3. Numeracy – calculation.

4. Neglect/inattention.

5. Dyspraxia.

6. Agnosia.

7. Graphaesthesia.

8. Astereoagnosis.

9. Two-point discrimination.

10. Right–left orientation.

In reality, the examiner would (thankfully) not expect you to examine all of these. Most likely, they will get you to focus on one particular aspect. For example, the examiner may say:

E – *This patient has a parietal lobe problem* (most likely this would be a volunteer patient - parietal lobe signs are not common). *Can you show me how you might elicit some of the signs of this?*

S – *The things I know about are graphaesthesia and astereognosis* (could also have said: two-point discrimination, arm drift [upwards and out]).

E – *Please examine for those.*

In relation to specific tests, the following are *brief* descriptions. If you are unsure, you will need to use one of the larger clinical skills/specialist textbooks.

Start with simply observing the patient. You may pick up strong clues of unilateral neglect or inattention in the way that the patient is sitting and ignoring one side of their body/space. There may be evidence of damage (bruising) to the affected side.

Language

Talk to the patient by introducing yourself and asking what the problem is. Listen carefully to their speech. An *expressive dysphasia* can be *non-fluent* speech indicating damage to the dominant (usually left) frontal hemisphere (Broca's area) or *fluent*, but non-sensical speech (Wernicke's area in tempero-parietal lobe). Can the patient understand very simple commands (without giving clues by gesture) such as 'open your eyes' (*receptive dysphasia*)?

If the patient seems to have difficulty in finding words, you should examine specifically for *nominal dysphasia*. Ask the patient to name some common object, such as a watch, then the parts (e.g. winder or strap).

Language also includes the ability to read (*dyslexia*) – get the person to read something from a newspaper or magazine (providing their vision is unimpaired). There may be problems with written communication (*dysgraphia*) – ask the patient to write a sentence (writing their name and address is too 'automatic' and is not the best test).

Ten-point mental test score

This is a standard test of mental function that you should be able to use in an OSCE station. The questions are:

1. Age
2. Time (to nearest hour)
3. Place
4. Address for recall at end of test. Patient should repeat the address to make sure that it has been heard correctly: *42 West Street*
5. Year
6. Recognition of two people (e.g. doctor, nurse, etc)
7. Date of birth (month and day sufficient)
8. Years of Second World War
9. Name of present monarch
10. Count backwards from 20 to 1.

Patients with no impairment will score at least 9/10.

EXAMINATION SKILLS

Numeracy

The ability to perform calculations can be affected by specific lesions in the dominant parietal lobe (angular gyrus) or, more commonly, the skill is lost as part of the global decline seen in dementias. The specific lesion may also affect right-left orientation and finger recognition (*Gerstmann–Straussler syndrome*). You should ask the patient to perform some simple sums, carry out 'serial 7s' (*'take 7 from 100 etc'*) and calculations involving money (*If I had £1.53 and bought a loaf of bread for 63p, how much would I have left?*).

Neglect/Inattention

This usually occurs (but not exclusively) in right hemisphere damage. The person shows less attention to one side of their body or space. Applying stimulation to both sides of the body at once will bring out mild problems (visual/sensory *extinction*). In severe forms, patients deny that one side of the body belongs to them. Pen and paper tests are very useful. Ask the patient to copy a flower, clock face or a house and observe whether they have not completed one side of the drawing. You can also draw multiple short lines on a piece of paper and ask the patient to cross out each of them (*cancellation test*).

Dyspraxia

Dyspraxia is the inability to carry out voluntary purposeful movement correctly (such as making a cup of tea) despite apparently normal motor, sensory and coordinative functions. It is usually seen in left cerebral hemisphere damage. Providing the patient can use their arm (not paralysed), ask them to show you how they would '*brush your teeth*' or '*strike a match*'.

Agnosia

Agnosia is a failure to recognise an object despite the sense by which it is normally recognised remaining intact (e.g. visual agnosia, sensory agnosia). This is different from nominal dysphasia where an object is recognised, but cannot be named. Agnosias occur with either left or right hemisphere damage. Ask the patient to name a pen, if they cannot do this, ask them to show you what to do with it. A patient with a nominal dysphasia cannot name a pen, but knows what it is used for. In agnosia, the person does not recognise the pen.

Graphaesthesia

The ability to interpret numbers written on the palm of the hand is located in the parietal lobe. It requires normal sensation in the hand. Ask the patient to hold out their hand and close their eyes. Tell them you are going to write a number on their palm and you want them to tell you what it is.

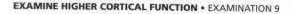

EXAMINATION SKILLS

ASTEREOAGNOSIS

A key function of the parietal lobe is to receive information from the sensory system and use this to tell the motor system what to do to obtain further sensory input. If you put an object, such as a key, in a person's hand, they will move it about, asking (unconsciously) such questions as *What is it made of, what shape is it, what are the edges like?*

Two-point discrimination

At the fingertips, a person has the ability to distinguish between two fine points 3–4 mm apart. This is lost early in a peripheral sensory neuropathy. However, if the sensory system is intact, the discrimination between one or two points is made in the parietal lobe. It is tested using a pair of dividers and asking the patient to close their eyes and indicate whether they *'feel one or two points'* as the dividers are moved further apart.

SUGGESTIONS FOR FURTHER PRACTICE

The only patients with consistent signs of language impairment or inattention are likely to be found in stroke rehabilitation units. You should also practise parts of the cognitive examination on any patients you see.

Extension to station (Level: ✱✱✱)

The most likely way that this station would be extended would be to include some examples of drawing tests showing inattention or constructional dyspraxia. Perseveration may also be demonstrated through drawing tests (e.g. a number will be repeated many times when 'drawing a clock face').

EXAMINATION 10 | # Vision

Level:	*
Setting:	Volunteer patient, being observed by examiner (may be truncated to use mannequin head). The following equipment is available to you: Snellen chart or near vision chart, torch, ophthalmoscope, large headed pin
Time:	5 min

TASK

E – *This person is complaining of problems with their vision. Please show me how you would examine this person's eyes.*

RESPONSE

The biggest pitfall in this station is to focus entirely on using an ophthalmoscope – particularly if the examiner hands you one! You need to break the examination into a number of sections according to the cranial nerves (II, III, IV, VI).

> **Core skill: Visual examination**
>
> The key steps are:
>
> 1. Test for visual acuity.
> 2. Test for visual fields.
> 3. Test for the light reflex.
> 4. Test for accommodation reflex.
> 5. Use the ophthalmoscope (included looking for the red reflex).
> 6. Test for eye movements.
> 7. Ask about diplopia.
> 8. Look for nystagmus.

Visual acuity

Test visual acuity *with each eye covered separately* using either the Snellen chart, near vision chart or a magazine/newspaper with the person wearing, and not wearing, glasses/contact lenses. You can grade visual loss at the bedside:

a. Can read ordinary type face
b. Can read newspaper headlines

EXAMINATION SKILLS

c. Can count fingers
d. Can see hand waving
e. Can distinguish between light and dark.

Visual fields

Test visual fields by confrontation using fingers in each of the four field quadrants. Test for *visual inattention* by using bilateral simultaneous stimulation. Find your blind spot by using a pin and, starting laterally, bringing it in slowly along the horizontal until it disappears and reappears. YOU *(and the patient) must keep looking straight ahead.*

Pupillary reflexes

Test for direct and indirect pupillary reflexes using pen torch. Examine and *comment on* shape, size and irregularity of pupil using the other eye to compare. Test for the accommodation reflex by asking the person to look at an object in the distance then *quickly* at your finger close to the nose (20–30 cm):

Look for:

- Convergence
- Slight ptosis
- Meiosis.

Using the ophthalmoscope

You always use your left eye to examine the patient's left eye and vice versa. This is hard but it is the accepted technique. Ideally you should keep your other eye open. It is alright to keep your own glasses on/lenses in – otherwise you have to correct the refractive error for both the patient and yourself.

With the lens setting at 0, and about 1 metre from the patient look through the aperture whilst shining the ophthalmoscope at the patient (partner) pupil. You should see a *red reflex* due to light reflecting from the back of the retina.

The patient should be asked to look into the distance – focus on a distant object. With your head and the ophthalmoscope forming a single unit, bring your eye slowly towards the patient's eye until you are as close as you can without touching. The back of the eye should be in focus. If not then adjust the lens keeping close to the patient. If the patient is short-sighted, a (minus – concave) lens should be tried in increasing strength. If long-sighted, a (positive – convex) lens is used.

You should follow a blood vessel back to the optic disc. Look at it – slightly pink with distinct margins. There should be four arteries (superior, inferior, nasal, temporal) with accompanying veins. Look at each – where they cross each other. Look at the surface of the retina. Examine for haemorrhages or exudates.

110

Lastly, look at the macula by asking the person to look directly at the light.

Eye movements

You are testing the III, IV and VI cranial nerves in unison. Look for (and *comment on*) strabismus (squint) – either convergent or divergent. Fix the head with one hand, then ask the patient to follow your finger with their eyes. Ask about seeing double at any stage. Use the 'H' pattern for individual muscles. Think about the rules of diplopia:

1. Diplopia maximum when looking in direction of impaired muscle
2. False image less distinct than true image
3. False image displaced furthest in the direction of action of impaired muscle.

Look for nystagmus (normal on extreme gaze):

1. Nystagmus named according to direction of fast movement
2. Always maximum when looking in direction of fast movement
3. Fast movement TOWARDS central lesion (e.g. cerebellum)
4. Fast movement AWAY peripheral lesion (e.g. vestibular apparatus).

SUGGESTIONS FOR FURTHER PRACTICE

Make a pact that you will examine the vision on all the patients you encounter in the next week, whether or not they have any visual problems.

Extensions to station (Levels: **/***)

There are many ways in which this station could be extended either by introducing a patient with visual problems or by showing you pictures after you have demonstrated your examination technique. The latter allows rarer (but very important) conditions to be included. The examiner may show you something then ask you what you would do next (e.g. in a patient with optic atrophy, a key investigation is magnetic resonance scanning because of demyelination).

Consider (and work on):

- Visual acuity problems – monocular blindness, multiple sclerosis
- Visual field loss – particularly homonymous hemianopia (common because of stroke)
- Abnormalities detectable on an ophthalmoscope:
  - Cataracts (very common)
  - Retinopathy (particularly diabetes)
  - Optic atrophy, papilloedema, hypertensive retinopathy (more likely as photographs or in a mannequin head)
  - Nystagmus
  - Oculomotor palsies (commonest VI nerve).

EXAMINATION SKILLS

EXAMINATION 11 — Hearing

Level:	*
Setting:	Volunteer patient (student). Sometimes mannequin heads are used with eardrum abnormalities. Available are: tuning fork, auroscope
Time:	5 min

TASK

E – *I would like you to show me how you would test hearing.*

RESPONSE

A test of hearing is not simply ascertaining whether the person is deaf, you must be able to demonstrate tuning fork tests and use of the auroscope.

Core skill: Examination of hearing

The key steps (in order) are:

1. Explain to a patient what you want to do
2. Test for any deafness.
3. Perform Rinne's test.
4. Perform Weber's test.
5. Use the auroscope.

Hearing

Test the hearing using a quiet whisper (repeat numbers) whilst rubbing the tragus of the opposite ear.

Tuning fork tests

Ideally the tuning fork should be 512 Hz – i.e. high pitched, not low pitched which is used for testing vibration.

Rinne's test
Test each ear independently. Strike the tuning fork and place it firmly on the bone behind the ear. Then place *in parallel* to the ear – with the tines vibrating toward the ear canal. Ask the patient which is the loudest. For a Rinne's positive

test the 2nd should be louder (air conduction > bone conduction). If the middle ear mechanism is damaged then BC > AC.

Weber's test

Strike the tuning fork and place it on the top of the head. It should be heard in the middle. Place a finger in one ear – the sound will become loudest there because of a temporary *conductive deafness*. In sensorineural deafness Weber's is *away* from the affected side. In conductive deafness it is *towards*.

Using the auroscope

Visually inspect the ear and canal before using the auroscope. The handle of the auroscope points towards the patient's nose and is held in the right hand when examining the patient's right ear. Use the biggest speculum possible, but one that fits easily into the external canal.

The external canal is bent slightly down and towards the patient's face. You have to straighten it by pulling up and back (*gently*) on the patient's ear with the hand not holding the auroscope. Then insert the auroscope and comment on the visibility and appearance of the drum.

SUGGESTIONS FOR FURTHER PRACTICE

The best place to learn about deafness is in an ENT or audiometry clinic. In a short time, you will see the examination clearly demonstrated (and probably have a chance to practice) and will come across the common abnormalities.

Extensions to station (Levels: **/***)

The station could be extended by

- Including a patient with deafness (very common, both sensorineural and conduction). The station would assess whether you could use Rinne's and Weber's test to correctly analyse the pattern.
- Using a mannequin head (or pictures) to illustrate various eardrum abnormalities. You should be able to recognise: perforation, otitis media (including bulging drum), grommets.
- Asking you to indicate what examination and investigation you would do if you suspected an acoustic neuroma (examination – corneal reflex, cerebellar–pontine angle – Vth, and VIIth nerve and coordination; investigation – MR scanning, audiometry).

EXAMINATION 12	**Examine the lower cranial nerves**
Level:	*
Setting:	Volunteer patient (student). Available are: glass of water, cotton wool, disposable pins
Time:	5 min

TASK

E – *Please show me how you would examine the cranial nerves, excluding smell, vision and hearing.*

RESPONSE

The instruction is quite complex. You have to stop and think what cranial nerves you need to test – V, VII, IX–XII nerves.

Core skill: Lower cranial nerve examination

You should test:

1. the Vth cranial nerve:
   - Motor
   - Sensory
   - Corneal reflex.

2. the VIIth cranial nerve:
   - Upper face
   - Lower face.

3. the IXth and Xth cranial nerves:
   - Motor
   - Swallowing.

4. the XIth cranial nerve.

5. the XIIth cranial nerve.

Vth cranial nerve (trigeminal)

Sensory

You need to test in each of the divisions of the trigeminal nerve (use the sternum to demonstrate the normal sensory stimuli):

- Light touch
- Pin-prick

- Corneal reflex: This is the most important sign to examine for if there is any question of trigeminal nerve damage. All reflexes have an afferent and an efferent arc, i.e. sensory – ophthalmic V; motor – facial VII.
  a. Ask the person to look up to the ceiling (thereby exposing the lower cornea).
  b. With a small wisp of cotton wool drawn to a point, lightly touch the lower cornea. You must not approach the eye directly as this will produce an aversion response. Approach from the side. The corneal reflex is quite unpleasant and should not be repeated several times! If impaired then the patient will not blink.

Motor

The muscles supplied by the trigeminal nerve are those of mastication (temporalis, masseters, and pterygoids).

- Examine for wasting – hollowing around the temporal arch.
- Ask the person to clench their teeth – you should be able to see the masseters and temporalis; palpate them to check their bulk.
- Ask them to open their mouth against resistance – this tests the pterygoids.
- Jaw jerk – sign of a bilateral upper motor nerve lesion above the level of the pons.

Ask the patient to lack their jaw open slightly. Place your index finger over the point of the jaw. With the patella hammer gently strike your finger in a downward motion. In a positive jaw jerk the muscles contract and the mouth will close.

Cranial nerve VII (facial)

The facial nerve is predominantly motor. Remember the bilateral innervation to the upper part of the face. So an **upper** motor neurone lesion will **spare** this. Look for (and *comment on*) any facial asymmetry. Mild facial weakness is best seen through flattening of the nasolabial fold.

Upper part of the face:

a. Furrow the brow
b. elevate the eyebrows
c. close the eyes.

Lower part of the face:

a. Blow out the cheeks
b. whistle
c. show teeth.

Cranial nerves IX (glossopharyngeal) and X (vagus)

The glossopharyngeal is predominantly sensory to the palate. It can be tested (if needed) through gently touching the pharyngeal arches on either side. The gag reflex is not a useful test (too variable in normal people).

EXAMINATION SKILLS

The vagus is predominantly motor. If there is palatal weakness, the patient will have a nasal quality to their speech.

- Ask the person to open their mouth and say 'aah'
- With a torch, and possibly a tongue depressor, observe the uvula. Does it lift centrally or is it pulled to one side (indicating weakness of the opposite side)?

A better test of cranial nerves IX and X is the coordinated act of swallowing:

1. Give the person a glass of water to drink.
2. Observe what happens – lip closure, elevation of the larynx, any spluttering/coughing (going down the 'wrong way').
3. Stand behind the person and place your fingers lightly on the larynx. Ask the person to swallow again. Feel for the elevation of the larynx.

Cranial nerve XI (accessory)

The accessory cranial nerve supplies sternomastoid and trapezius.

1. Observe for wasting.
2. Ask the person to push their head forward against your hand – it will make the sternomastoid contract.
3. Request that they turn their head sideways against your hand – it will make the opposite sternomastoid contract.
4. Ask the person to shrug their shoulders – observe for elevation of trapezius.

Cranial nerve XII (hypoglossal)

1. Ask the person to open their mouth.
2. Using a torch, inspect the tongue for wasting and fasciculation.
3. Ask the person to put their tongue out – it will point towards the side of any weakness.

Extensions to station (Levels: **/***)

The commonest cranial nerve abnormality is a facial weakness. You must be able to distinguish (and clearly explain) the difference between an upper and lower facial nerve lesion (see above).

EXAMINATION 13 — Examine the sensory system in the arms

Level:	*
Setting:	Volunteer patient (student). Available are: some disposable neurological pins, cotton wool and a tuning fork
Time:	5 min

TASK

E – *Please show me how you would test sensation in this person's upper limbs.*

RESPONSE

Practice your examination and rate yourself (or get your partner to do so) according to the steps listed in the core skill box. The examiner would have a mark sheet based on this and would either 'tick a box' as you performed each step or use the criteria to give you an overall mark.

Core skill: Sensory examination of the arms

The key steps are:

1. Give clear instructions to the patient during the examination.

2. Show awareness of how to test sensation in dermatomal/nerve distribution.

3. Test vibration sense appropriately.

4. Test pin-prick sensation.

5. Test proprioception.

6. Test light touch.

7. Summarise your findings for the examiner.

You must know the dermatomes and sensory distribution of the major nerves to examine sensation and interpret your findings (see Fig. 4.3). The main sensory modalities tested are:

- Pin-prick – superficial pain
- Vibration
- Joint position – proprioception
- Light touch.

Note that light touch comes last. The reason for this is it is the most difficult to do well and interpret correctly. Examine the arms separately working through all

EXAMINATION SKILLS

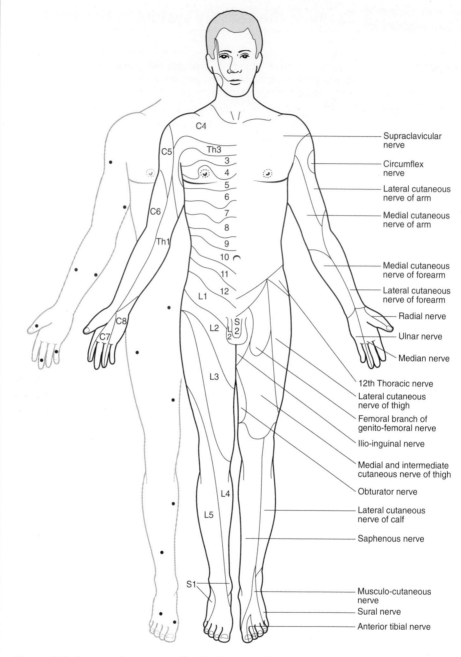

Figure 4.3 Sensory dermatome distribution over the anterior surface of the body. The points illustrate the most efficient places to test for sensory disturbance within dermatomes

the modalities. Make sure that the patient holds his arms in the anatomical position (palms uppermost).

Pin-prick

For pin-prick use disposable neurological pins. Do *not* use the standard venepuncture needles. These are designed to puncture the skin to take blood – it is not good to leave the patient covered with drops of blood! Demonstrate the sensation to the patient over the sternum. Say to the patient *This is sharp; This is blunt; Please shut your eyes and say blunt or sharp when you feel the pin.*

Test the patient's ability to feel the sensation in each of the dermatomes (C4 shoulder–T2 chest wall). Also consider the nerves of the hand. If there is any abnormality, delineate the loss by moving from the centre of the area of loss/impairment to the normal area.

Vibration

The principals are:

- You must not have the tuning fork (128 Hz) vibrating audibly
- You must apply the tuning fork firmly over a bony prominence.

You can check that the person is feeling the vibration and not the cold metal by getting them to close their eyes and applying the tuning fork either vibrating or not. Similarly, you can ask the person to indicate when the vibration stops – do this by touching the tines of the tuning fork. In the hands, test this first over the nail beds, then at the wrist, elbow and finally the sternum.

Joint position sense

The most important principals about testing joint position sense are:

- Demonstrate what you want to the patient with their eyes open. *'This movement is up, this movement is down – I want you to say up or down when you detect any movement.'*
- Make sure that you grasp the finger at the *sides* so that you do not give an indication of movement through pressure.
- Use fine not gross movements – try it on yourself at the fingers.

You start with the most distal joint (DIP) and move proximally until the sensation is detected.

Light touch

This is the most difficult sensation to test, because the patients find it very difficult to indicate consistently changes/abnormality. You must:

- Use a fine touch not a tickling or stroking movement.

EXAMINATION SKILLS

- Ask the patient to close their eyes and simply say yes or no as to when they feel something.

As with pin-prick, you should test in the middle of each dermatome. If you find that the patient has sensory loss in a T1/T2 distribution (medial border of arms), you should test sensation over the trunk to determine a lower level (if present):

T2   2nd interspace
T8   Costal margin
T10 Umbilicus
T12 Pubic symphysis.

SUGGESTIONS FOR FURTHER PRACTICE

As with Examination 15 (Examine the motor system in the arms). Apart from neurological departments, consider going to orthopaedic, plastic surgery (hand) or minor injury units ('cuts/lacerations' require the doctor to check out that there has not been any nerve damage – this gives you an opportunity to practise). Diabetes units will have patients with peripheral neuropathies. Patients with strokes often have gross sensory loss (hemisensory anaesthesia).

Extensions to station (Level: ✱✱✱)

Peripheral neuropathies tend to involve the feet first (see Examination 14), but you could encounter someone with a 'glove' loss. More common would be a patient with a carpal tunnel syndrome or (less frequent) an ulnar nerve palsy (see Examination 15 extensions).

EXAMINATION 14	**Sensory examination**
Level:	**
Setting:	Examine a patient with a peripheral neuropathy (e.g. diabetic)
Time:	10 min

TASK

E – *This patient is complaining that they 'feel that they are walking on cotton wool'. Please examine the sensation in their legs, I will then ask you to present your findings.*

RESPONSE

The examiner will observe you performing the examination. At the end, you need to tell them what you have found. There is a large clue to what you will find from the phrase 'walking on cotton wool'. This is highly suggestive of a peripheral neuropathy, so you should be examining with this to the forefront. You might also look for injection sites consistent with diabetes.

E – *So, what have you found?*

S – *There seems to be a total loss of sensation from the mid-calf down on the left on the right and from the knee down on the left. Above this, the patient could feel things, but said that the sensation was queer.*

E – *I noticed that you started with pin-prick. Why did you do that?*

S – *I find that this is easier to get the patient to understand what I am doing and how they should respond.*

E – *Why not light touch?*

S – *I used to do that, but I found that it confused me, with a lot of patients their answers were not clear.*

E – *What did you find with vibration sense.*

S – *It was absent below the pelvis.*

E – *If you were unsure whether the patient was detecting vibration as opposed to the coldness of the metal, is there anything you could do?*

S – *I don't know of any different method.*

E – *Well, you could get the patient to close their eyes and tell you whether they can feel the vibration. If they say yes, ask them to tell you when it stops. You can then touch the tuning fork to stop it and see if the patient responds quickly – or still says that the fork is vibrating. So, what do you think the diagnosis is?*

S – *Most likely, it is a peripheral neuropathy causing a stocking loss.*

E – *But it is more on the left than the right.*

S – *I don't think that it has to be perfectly symmetrical.*

E – *That's right. What is the most likely underlying problem?*

S – *Probably diabetes mellitus.*

E – *Fine, there's the bell.*

EXAMINATION SKILLS

For more detail on sensory testing see Examination 13.

Core skill: Sensory examination of the legs

1. Know the dermatomes and important nerve innervation of the legs.

2. The main sensory modalities tested are:
   - Pin-prick – superficial pain
   - Vibration (ankle, knee, pelvis)
   - Joint position – proprioception (big toe, ankle)
   - Light touch (last).

3. Stand the patient up (if possible) and then ask them to walk (see Table 4.3, page 131).

4. Romberg's test: Ask the patient to stand with feet slightly apart. If they sway with their eyes closed, this is a sign of posterior column disease (Romberg's test is *positive*).

SUGGESTIONS FOR FURTHER PRACTICE

In the diabetic clinic, patients will have regular assessments of the feet including general foot care, blood supply and evidence of peripheral neuropathy. Go along and practise!

Extension to station (Level: ***)

In sensory testing, you have to put the patterns together. In the legs, the most likely problem is a stocking loss due to a peripheral neuropathy (diabetes). Occasionally, you will see patients with root lesions (particularly L5). Occasionally, patients have differential loss of sensation, e.g. loss of joint position and vibration in posterior column damage due to B_{12} deficiency.

EXAMINATION 15 — Examine the motor system in the arms

Level:	**/***
Setting:	A patient in a wheelchair (see Fig. 4.4). A tendon hammer is available
Time:	10 min

TASK

E – *This patient is complaining of difficulty in using his arms. Please show me how you would examine the motor system in this person's upper limbs. I would like you to discuss your findings as you go along.*

RESPONSE

This station involves a real patient, which requires a different approach to working through the task. If you look at the picture, you can see that the left arm is held across the body. This strongly suggests that the patient's arm is paralysed. A monoparesis of an arm is most likely to be due to an upper motor lesion. Apart from trauma, most lower motor neurone palsies would not affect the whole arm or, if they did, would affect the other arm as well (see below).

> **Core skill: Examining real patients**
>
> In this task, there are two crucial aspects:
>
> 1. **You must spend time observing.** This is not simply to get the 'point' for being seen to do so, but because there may be strong clues to the diagnosis, which allow you to plan your examination efficiently and effectively.
>
> 2. The examiner has told you to talk through the examination. This is so that they can assess whether you are appreciating what you are eliciting in your examination and can put the signs together into a diagnosis.

An upper motor neurone weakness is likely to lead to:

- Increased tone (compare with other side)
- Increased reflexes
- Weakness – particularly of triceps, finger extensors, and hand grip (giving the typical posture).

Remember the instruction to 'Discuss your findings'. You should be clear in your response to this and how you are interpreting the signs.

S – *Comparing the reflexes, I think that there is a generalised increase on the left*

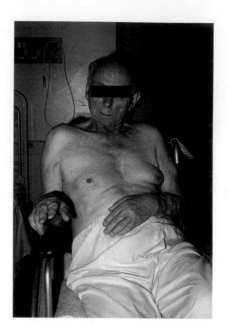

Figure 4.4

side compared to the right. This would be in keeping with the increased tone on the left.

E – *Given the brisk jerks, are there any other reflexes that you could examine in the upper limb?*

S – *You could look for a finger jerk.*

E – *Show me.*

S – *I would ask the patient to flex his fingers around mine like this. I would then strike the extensor aspects of my fingers, producing a brief extension of the patient's fingers. With a positive jerk – like this – what you see is a reflex flexion of the fingers and movement of the thumb across the palm.*

E – *Very good.*

General aspects of neurological examination of the arms

Inspection

- As you start your examination, you should look for any obvious problems: abnormal movements (tremor – rest or intentional, chorea – jerking random movements and athetosis – slow writhing movements), or not using one arm.
- Expose the arms: look for wasting around the shoulders/upper arms (proximal) and hands (distal) – you need to look at both the palmar and dorsal surfaces. Is any wasting symmetrical or localised?
- Look for *fasciculation*, which is intermittent twitching of muscle fibres (particularly deltoid and the first dorsal interossei muscle) – it is a sign of subacute denervation (motor neurone disease).

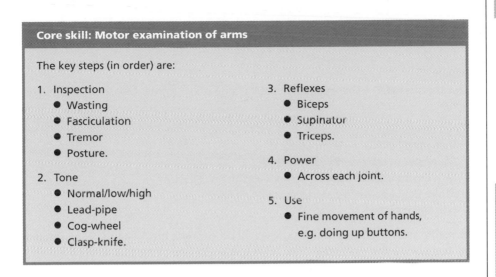

Tone

It is best to test tone and reflexes *before* power – this stops the patient 'helping' you by performing movements actively.

- Holding the arm at the wrist move it across two joints (elbow, wrist) simultaneously in a random manner.
- Tone can be normal, low or increased – compare with the other side. Low tone is difficult to assess.
- *Clasp-knife (spasticity)* is best brought out by rapid movement (upper motor neurone).
- *Lead-pipe (cog-wheel)* is best brought out by slow movement (extra-pyramidal).

Reflexes

You *must* use the long-handled tendon hammer. The technique involves letting the hammer fall under its own weight onto the tendon – you direct it rather than add force. Ask the patient to rest their arms loosely over their abdomen/lower chest with one arm on top of the other. Test the following reflexes:

- **Biceps (C5):** Place your thumb over the biceps tendon and strike this with the hammer – watch for elbow flexion.
- **Supinator (C6):** Strike the supinator tendon on the lateral side of the forearm just above the wrist – watch for elbow extension and muscle contraction.
- **Triceps (C7):** Strike the triceps tendon just above the elbow on the posterior surface – watch for elbow extension and muscle contraction.

Reflexes can be normal, increased, reduced or absent. Note the pattern for each reflex. The usual reason for apparent absence is poor technique. If they appear to be absent – you must employ *'reinforcement'* – this temporarily increases muscle tone. Ask the patient to 'clench your teeth' just as you are about to hit

the tendon. This will increase the strength of the reflex obtained and may make it visible.

Power

Test the strength of the muscles across all the major joints. Use the MRC power scale:

0 No movement
1 Just a flicker of muscle movement
2 Movement with gravity eliminated
3 Movement against gravity, but not against resistance
4 Movement against resistance but not normal
5 Normal power.

In reality, most people with weakness will lie between grade 4 and 5 – evaluate it by comparing the two sides. You 'eliminate' gravity by testing movement in a horizontal plane. As a quick screen, test for:

- Shoulder – abduction/adduction
- Elbow and wrist – flexion/extension
- Fingers – flexion/abduction.

You need to know the major myotomes moving across these joints:

Shoulder abduction	C4
Shoulder adduction	C5
Elbow flexion	C6
Elbow extension	C7
Finger flexion	C8
Finger abduction	T1

Extensions to station (Levels: **/***)

The other common motor abnormalities affecting the upper limbs are the mononeuropathies:

- **Median:** Wasting of thenar eminence. Test for abductor pollicis brevis (APB) and opponens policis. Also tell the examiner that you would test for sensory loss (thumb, index, middle and half of ring finger).
- **Ulnar:** Wasting of interossei (look at 1st between thumb and index) and hypothenar eminence. Test for adductor pollicis (Froment's sign), finger abduction/adduction and abduction of little finger. State you would test for sensory loss (little finger half of ring).

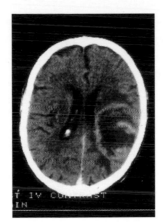

Figure 4.5

- **Radial:** No wasting of hand. If high lesion (axilla – due to 'crutch' palsy or invasion by tumour) – triceps weak. Not the case if 'Saturday night palsy' – pressure on nerve in spiral groove of humerus. Comment on wrist drop. You should demonstrate weakness of wrist and finger extension. Test other muscles of hand by fixing wrist on hard flat surface. Minimal sensory loss, may be none or confined to skin over 1st dorsal interosseus.

The station could also be linked to data:

E – *If I tell you that the upper motor signs in the left arm have been coming on over several weeks, how would that influence your differential diagnosis?*
S – *It would strongly suggest a space occupying lesion.*
E – *So what would you do next?*
S – *I would request a CT scan of the head.*
E – *Here is the CT scan. How do you interpret it?*

(see Fig. 4.5).

The scan is taken after the administration of intravenous contrast. It shows a large irregular enhancing lesion in the right temperoparental region with some surrounding oedema. There is no mid-line shift, but there is some compression of the lateral ventricle. It is either a primary glioma or a large metastasis.

SUGGESTIONS FOR FURTHER PRACTICE

Apart from neurology clinics, the other areas of the hospital where patients with neurological abnormalities affecting upper limbs can be found are: orthopaedic clinics (carpal tunnel, ulnar nerve entrapment at elbow, spine – disc protrusion), stroke rehabilitation units, plastic surgery clinics (hand problems).

EXAMINATION SKILLS

EXAMINATION 16	**Examine the motor system in the legs**
Level:	***
Setting:	A patient standing by a couch
Time:	10 min

TASK

E – *This patient is complaining of difficulty in walking. Please show me how you would examine the motor system in the lower limbs.*

(See Fig. 4.6).

RESPONSE

Look at the patient. You should ask yourself:

- What is the position of the legs and feet? Is either foot in plantar-flexion (suggesting a foot-drop that you can formally examine for)?
- Is there any evidence of foot deformity (e.g. pes cavus – Friedreich's ataxia)?
- Is there any wasting either proximally and distally? Is any wasting symmetrical or localised?
- Is there *fasciculation*, which can be normal in the calf?

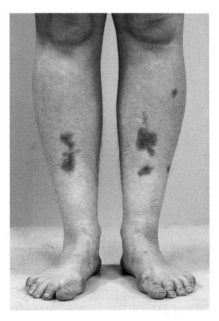

Figure 4.6

Core skill: Motor examination of the legs

1. Inspection:
   - Position
   - Wasting
   - Fasciculation
   - Deformity.

2. Tone:
   - Roll the leg on the bed and test for clonus.

3. Reflexes:
   - Test the knee (L3, L4)
   - Test the ankle (L5, S1)
   - Test the plantar response.

4. Power:
   - Test the strength of the muscles across all the major joints. Use the MRC power scale.

5. Gait:
   - If able, ask the patient to walk.

In this case, the photograph shows two abnormalities:

- Flat feet (pes planus)
- Necrobiosis lipoidica diabeticorum.

Together, these suggest that you are faced with a patient who has a peripheral neuropathy due to diabetes. You can then examine the patient on the couch, looking for:

- Distal weakness
- Loss of ankle and, possibly, knee jerks
- Symmetry in terms of abnormalities (may be some inequality, but both sides will be affected)
- You must (in any examination of the motor system in the lower limbs) assess walking (see below), **providing** that the patient indicates that they are able to do so and you judge it safe from your examination of them on the couch
- You can indicate to the examiner that you would expect a 'stocking' sensory loss.

General examination of motor system in legs

Inspection

See above.

Tone

You can test tone in one of three ways:

1. Roll the leg on the bed (internal/external rotation of the hip).

EXAMINATION SKILLS

2. Place your hand under the knee and lift up suddenly to approximately 10 cm. Usually the heel will lift and fall back on the bed. If high tone – heel stays off bed. If low tone heel does not rise from the bed.
3. Flex and extend the knee.

Reflexes

Test the knee (L3, L4), ankle (L5, S1) and plantar response. For the *knee jerk*, place your arm under the patient's knees (both together) and lift them to approximately 20° flexion with the heels on the bed and the quadriceps relaxed. Let the hammer fall on the patellar tendon just below the patella. Watch for quadriceps contraction and knee extension.

For the *ankle jerk*, get the patient to abduct the hip slightly, flex the knee and let it fall outwards. One hand grasps the forefoot and adjusts the tone in the calf muscles by altering the amount of dorsi-flexion. The hammer is allowed to fall onto the Achilles tendon. Watch for plantar flexion and calf muscle contraction.

The two commonest faults in demonstrating the ankle reflex are:

- not having the leg/foot in the right position
- not having the right amount of tone in the calf muscles.

If any of the reflexes appear absent then apply *reinforcement* by getting the patient to interlock their fingers and asking them to pull as you strike the hammer.

Plantar response

Say to the patient 'I am now going to scrape the bottom of your foot' (not 'tickle'). With the sharp end of the tendon hammer, scrape along the outside of the foot from the heel towards the toes and then across the forefoot. Watch the toes.

- The normal response is for the big toe (and the others) to plantar flex (plantar down-going).
- The abnormal response is for the big toe to extend (dorsiflex) and the other toes to fan (plantar up-going).

Power

As with the upper limb, you need to test the strength of the muscles across all the major joints. Use the MRC power scale. You need to know the major myotomes moving across these joints:

Hip adduction	L1–3
Hip abduction	L3
Hip flexion	L3, L4
Hip extension	L4, L5
Knee flexion	L4, L5
Knee extension	L3, L4
Dorsiflexion of foot	L5
Plantar flexion of foot	S1

Gait

At some stage you should see the patient walk if they are able to do so.

- Do they limp?
- Are they unsteady?
- Do they hold onto things?
- Do they appear stiff (spastic)?
- Do they have foot drop?
- Do their arms swing when they walk?

SUGGESTIONS FOR FURTHER PRACTICE

Apart from neurological out-patient clinics, you might spend time on a 5 day unit where patients with neurological problems are often admitted for investigation. Many centres also run specialist services for patients with Parkinson's disease.

Extensions to station (Levels: **/***)

There are a number of different ways that this station could be extended using common neurological problems:

- A patient with a hemiparesis (as with Examination station 15)
- A patient with bilateral upper motor neurone signs (such as multiple sclerosis)
- A patient with Parkinson's disease
- A patient with ataxia (see Examination station 17) or other gait disturbance (see Table 4.3).

Table 4.3 Gait disturbance

Gait description	Interpretation
Flexed posture, *loss of arm swing*, small steps, centre of gravity leaning forward, difficulty in stopping, changing direction to command	Parkinson's disease
Arm may be flexed and adducted across body (no arm swing). Leg is extended with circumduction when the patient has to swing the leg around (cannot flex the knee – foot would catch on floor if leg brought straight through)	Hemiparesis (stroke)
Wide-based posture (sway with eyes open). Needs to hold on to furniture (you) to walk	Cerebellar disease
High-stepping gait on that side to prevent the foot catching as person brings leg through. Foot drop can be observed (lesser degrees brought out by asking patient to stand on heels)	Foot drop (Lateral popliteal palsy)
High-stepping 'stomping' gait as patient is unaware of position of feet. Very careful as they walk – no feedback	Peripheral neuropathy (Joint position sense)
Painful gait (antalgic). Does not want to weight bear through the affected joint. Quickly steps through to transfer weight through other leg	Arthritis

In relation to bilateral upper motor neurone signs, the examiner may ask:

E – *You have commented on the general increase in tone, is there any other sign you might want to look for?*
S – *I would look for clonus.*
E – *Show me.*
S – *I would grasp the forefoot like this, and tell the patient that I am going to move it quite quickly, but that it will not hurt. I would then dorsiflex it and hold the foot in this position. This is true clonus as it keeps going as long as I hold the foot in position.*
E – *When you had finished examining the legs, is there anything else you would want to do?*
S – *I would like to examine the arms.*

Patients with **Parkinson's disease** are also readily available to the examiners and will have stable signs. You could encounter such a patient through:

- Examination of someone with a tremor (contrasting with benign essential tremor – **positional**, bilateral, symmetrical, often mild, and worsened by emotion – ask about family history).
- Mask-like facies.
- 'Gait' station - see Table 4.3.

In your approach to the examination of someone with possible Parkinson's disease, think about:

Tremor

Coarse (4–6 Hz) affecting the thumb and fingers; as the disease progresses it may worsen to affect the hand, arm and trunk (and other side, but often **asymmetrical** – as with other signs). It disappears during complete relaxation/sleep and is made worse by holding a posture and by anxiety.

Bradykinesia and rigidity

Slowness and difficulty in initiating and changing any voluntary movement. Accompanying the bradykinesia, is an increase in tone. This rigidity is present throughout passive movement of a limb – *lead-pipe* (c.f. the 'clasp-knife' increase in tone seen in pyramidal tract disorders). The superimposition of the tremor on the hypertonia leads to *cog-wheel rigidity*.

Posture

Flexed with a shuffling gait (*festinant*).

Other features are loss of facial expression, dysphagia and dribbling of saliva. The voice is reduced in amplitude (*dysphonia*) with little intonation and a tendency to peter out.

EXAMINATION 17	**Examine coordination**
Level:	***
Setting:	A young patient with incoordination sitting in a wheelchair
Time:	10 min

TASK

E – *This patient feels that they are becoming more clumsy. Please show me how you would test coordination in the patient.*

RESPONSE

The examiner is telling you that the patient has difficulty with coordination. The core skill is set out in the box.

> **Core skill: Coordination**
>
> 1. Ascertain which is the patient's dominant hand and make allowances for the relative lack of coordination in the other hand.
> 2. In the arms, perform at least one of the following:
>   - Finger–nose test
>   - Disdiadochokinesis (rapid alternative hand movements)
>   - Fine finger movements.
> 3. Perform heel–shin test.
> 4. Ask if you can stand the patient up.
> 5. Perform Romberg's test.
> 6. Ask if you can observe the patient walking.

In neurological examination, the last modality to be tested is coordination as this requires intact sensory and motor systems. Usually problems with coordination are due to cerebellar disease. Always ask the patient which is their dominant hand and make allowances for the relative lack of coordination of the other hand.

Arms

In the arms there are a number of tests of coordination:

1. *Finger–nose:* Hold your index finger about 50 cm away from the patient's nose. Ask the patient to use the index finger of one hand to touch your finger,

then their nose, and repeat it as fast as they can. You can move your own hand a little to make the test harder. Ask the patient to repeat it with the other hand.

In a patient with cerebellar disease, you may see *intention tremor or past pointing* – as the patient gets closer to the target their finger does not home in on it, but starts to oscillate more and more and often overshoots.

2. *Rapid alternating hand movements (disdiadochokinesis):* Ask the patient to tap the back of one of their hands with the other, alternating with the palm and the back of the hand. Can they do this rapidly? Are there any differences between the two sides?

3. *Fine finger movements:* Ask the patient to touch each finger in turn with their thumb. Is this clumsy, are there differences between the two sides?

Legs

In the legs, demonstrate the *heel–shin test*. Ask the patient to lift one leg off the bed, place the heel on the knee of the other leg and run it down the shin and finally lift it in the air to touch your finger with their big toe. Again, compare the two sides to get an idea of any impairment.

Truncal ataxia

Finally, stand the patient up if they can do so unsupported.

Romberg's test

Ask the patient to stand with their eyes open and feet slightly apart. If they have marked sway with their eyes open, this indicates cerebellar disease. Ask the patient to close their eyes – if the sway appears now, this is a sign of posterior column disease (Romberg's test is *positive*).

Observe the patient walking (Table 4.3) – a patient with midline (vermis) cerebellar damage will have gross truncal ataxia, very unsteady and will walk with a wide-based gait.

SUGGESTIONS FOR FURTHER PRACTICE

Neurology clinics, programmed investigation and neurological rehabilitation units are the most likely areas that you will see patients with coordination problems. A small number of patients with stroke have cerebellar signs, but this is uncommon.

Extension to station (Level: ***)

Having observed you demonstrating that the patient has major coordination problems, the examiner may ask:

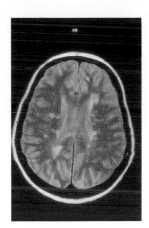

Figure 4.7

E – *Is there anything else you would like to examine for?*
S – *I would look for nystagmus.*
E – *Why?*
S – *It would help to confirm that the cerebellum is involved.*
E – *What do you think the diagnosis is?*
S – *Well, the person is quite young, so I would consider an inherited problem such as Friedreich's ataxia and carefully ask about family history.*
E – *There is no significant family history.*
S – *I would think that the likely diagnosis is multiple sclerosis.*
E – *Could you tell me what you think about this magnetic resonance (MR) scan (Fig. 4.7).*
S – *It shows multiple small white areas around the ventricles and throughout the brain.*
E – *How do you interpret these?*
S – *In multiple sclerosis, you get plaques throughout the central white matter.*
E – *Excellent.*

Patients with multiple sclerosis (MS) are readily accessible for OSCE organisers. As well as coordination, they could be included in the examination because of visual impairment (optic atrophy) and upper motor neurone signs. The diagnosis of MS is made on two episodes of neurological impairment different in both time and area of the brain affected. MR is the first-line investigation in suspected MS. Multiple plaques of demyelination occur in the periventricular white matter, cerebellum, optic pathways, spinal cord and brain stem. Acute plaques can enhance with gadolinium.

EXAMINATION 18	Lymph node examination
Level:	**
Setting:	A normal volunteer (student)
Time:	5 min

TASK

E – *Show me how you would examine for lymphadenopathy in this patient. Exclude the groins in your examination.*

RESPONSE

The examiner wants you to be able to consider where you might palpate for enlarged lymph nodes and then demonstrate how you might do this.

Core skill: Lymph node examination

1. Examine for lymphadenopathy in the following lymph node fields:
   - Cervical
   - Supraclavicular
   - Infraclavicular
   - Epitrochlear
   - Axillary
   - Para-aortic

2. If you find any enlargement, consider: size, consistency, tenderness, fixation and overlying skin tethering or discolouration.

This station is likely to cause a lot of anxiety because it requires you to cut across the usual examination of the body by system. If you feel any lymph node enlargement, you should consider:

- Size: anything greater than 1 cm are abnormal
- Consistency: Hardness suggests carcinoma, a rubbery consistency points to lymphoma
- Tenderness: implies infection
- Fixation: Suggests malignancy
- Overlying skin: tethering is a feature of malignancy, inflammation suggests infection.

Cervical

You should examine the patient from behind and with the patient sitting up. In total, there are seven groups. Start with the *submental* node just under the chin, then move your fingers to just below the angle of the jaw (*sub-mandibular*). Next, feel for the *jugular chain* which lies anterior to the sternomastoid muscle and then the *posterior triangle* nodes which are posterior to the sternomastoid muscle. Palpate the *occipital* region and then the *post-auricular* and the *pre-auricular* node in front of the ear.

Supraclavicular

From the front, palpate for nodes in the supraclavicular fossa and at the base of the sternocleidomastoid muscle.

Infraclavicular

The infraclavicular nodes can be palpated just beneath the clavicle.

Epitrochlear

These are palpated at the elbow. Place the palm of your left hand under the patient's left elbow. Your thumb can then palpate proximal and slightly anterior to the medial epicondyle.

Axillary

Lift up the patient's arm, then using your left hand palpate for axillary nodes in the right axilla (and vice versa for the left axilla). Push your finger tips towards the apex of the axilla. There are five groups corresponding to a four-sided pyramid: *apical/central, lateral, pectoral (medial), anterior and posterior*.

Para-aortic

A deep central mass can occasionally be due to enlarged para-aortic nodes.

Remember to complete the examination of the lymphatic system by stating (or demonstrating) that you would examine for hepatosplenomegaly.

SUGGESTIONS FOR FURTHER PRACTICE

Patients with stable lymphadenopathy are relatively uncommon. However, lymph node examination is part of the routine screen in breast, oncology and haematology clinics.

Extension to station (Level: ***)

The easiest way to extend the station would be to ask you to discuss further

EXAMINATION SKILLS

investigation. This would commonly involve showing you images such as hilar lymphadenopathy on a chest radiograph or possibly a CT scan.

Definitive investigation requires biopsy. If you are shown a biopsy report (or histology section) remember that it most likely shows either lymphoma or carcinoma. The history that the examiner gives would be very helpful (e.g. a 27-year-old person is much more likely to have Hodgkin's lymphoma than carcinoma).

EXAMINATION 19 — Examine the neck

Level:	***
Setting:	A patient sitting on a chair
Time:	5 min

TASK

E – *What do you notice about this patient's neck?*
S – *There is a swelling over the anterior part.*
E – *What do you think it is?*
S – *Judging from its position, I would say that it is a goitre.*
E – *Before I ask you to examine the neck, if you thought the thyroid gland was underactive, what questions might you ask of the patient?*
S – *You could ask about cold intolerance, or dryness of skin, change in voice.*
E – *Now can you please examine this patient's thyroid gland.*

RESPONSE

Patients with goitres (particularly multinodular) are quite common, so quite complex OSCE stations can be built around thyroid disease (hyper/hypothyroid or euthyroid).

Core skill: Examination of thyroid gland

1. Explain to the patient what you want to do.

2. Uncover the neck adequately and accurately describe the appearance of any goitre.

3. Give the patient a glass of water, and ask him/her to swallow. Comment on what you observe.

4. Examine the goitre and neck from behind the patient. Comment on shape, consistency, tenderness and nodularity of the thyroid.

5. Palpate for thyroid movement on swallowing (fixed or mobile).

6. Examine for lymphadenopathy.

7. Listen for bruits (vascularity).

The steps in neck examination are:

Inspection

Look at the front and side of the neck to decide whether there is a localised or general swelling of the gland. Ask the patient to take a sip of water and watch the swelling when the patient swallows. Only a goitre or a thyroglossal cyst will rise on swallowing (because of attachment to the larynx). Rarely, a thyroid neoplasm will invade the surrounding tissues and prevent movement. It is also important to look for any scars from previous surgery.

Palpation

You should examine the patient from behind. Use both hands and examine using the pulps of your finger tips. Systematically palpate both lobes and the central isthmus. You should comment on:

- Size: particularly feel for a lower border (many goitres have retrosternal extensions).
- Shape: is the gland uniformly enlarged or irregular (nodular)? If there is a solitary nodule, note its size, consistency, location and whether it is fixed.
- Consistency: the gland may feel firm in a simple goitre. A stony hard nodule suggests carcinoma.
- Tenderness: is a sign of thyroiditis.
- Mobility: neoplastic infiltration may fix the gland.

You should repeat the assessment as the patient swallows. As part of palpation, you should examine for cervical lymphadenopathy (carcinoma).

Auscultation

A bruit is a sign of increased blood supply and occasionally is heard in thyro-toxicosis.

At the end of the examination of a goitre, the examiner may ask you to state, or examine for, other signs of hypo- or hyperthryoidism.

E – *If you thought that the patient was hypothyroid, what else would you want to examine?*

- General cognitive slowness on talking to patient
- Cool and dry skin
- Bradycardia
- Alopecia/thinning of scalp hair
- 'Croaking' speech
- Delayed relaxation of ankle jerks (classically demonstrated at ankle, but easily brought out with the supinator jerks).

Signs of thyrotoxicosis include

- Sympathetic overactivity: tremor, tachycardia, sweating.
- Onycholysis (separation of the nail from its bed)
- Thyroid acropachy (looks like clubbing)

- Palmar erythema
- Proximal myopathy
- Lid retraction.

Graves' eye disease

- Exophthalmos (examine from behind and above – the eyes should not be visible beyond the supra-orbital ridge)
- Complications of the proptosis:
  - Chemosis
  - Conjunctivitis
  - Corneal ulceration
  - Ophthalmoplegia.

SUGGESTION FOR FURTHER PRACTICE

Patients with goitres/eye signs are relatively common in general medicine, even when these are not the problems the patient has been admitted/come to clinic about. However, the best place to see active disease is in the endocrinology/thyroid clinic.

Extension to station

A different station could involve a patient with proptosis from previous Graves' disease. Any station focussed on thyroid disease is likely to include asking you for interpretation of thyroid function tests.

EXAMINATION SKILLS

EXAMINATION 20	Examine the spine
Level:	*
Setting:	A normal volunteer standing by a couch
Time:	5 min

TASK

E – *This patient has a problem with the spine, please show me the appropriate examination.*

RESPONSE

This is a straightforward station providing you have learnt how to examine the spine.

Core skill: Examination of the spine

1. Observe and comment on any deformity.

2. Feel and percuss for tenderness over each vertebral body.

3. Feel and percuss for sacroiliac tenderness.

4. Examine for active movement:
   - Flexion
   - Extension
   - Lateral bending
   - Rotation.

5. Ask the patient to demonstrate straight leg raising.

6. Observe the patient walking.

The reason most students find examination of the spine difficult is that they have not practised the examination very much. However, it can be broken down into what you might observe and then what movements occur at the spine.

Observation may confirm the normal thoracic kyphosis and lumbar lordosis. You should look for exaggeration of kyphosis (may be due to osteoporosis in elderly people) and scoliosis (trauma, vertebral body disease, developmental abnormalities, or muscle problems).

Tenderness over a vertebral body is a very important sign that separates sinister from non-sinister back disease. You should consider metastatic disease, infection or collapse. Tenderness over the sacroiliac joints is indicative of a sero-negative spondylo-arthropathy.

- *Flexion* of the spine is assessed by asking the patient to touch their toes with the knees straight.
- *Extension* is tested by requesting the patient to lean backwards.
- *Lateral bending* – get the patient to slide their left hand as far down their left leg as possible, repeating the test on the other side. This movement is affected early in ankylosing spondylitis.
- *Rotation* – sit the patient on a stool (or fix the pelvis from behind) and ask the patient to rotate their head and shoulders as far as they can.

Straight leg raising is limited by pain in lower lumbar disc prolapse (L3, L4 prolapse causes restriction in hip extension).

SUGGESTIONS FOR FURTHER PRACTICE

Success in this station will come through looking as though you have done a spinal examination before! Practice with your colleagues so that it runs smoothly without long pauses whilst you think!

Extensions to station (Level: ***)

Most commonly, the station will involve going through spinal examination on a normal patient. However, if a patient is used, then most likely the spinal disease will be due to ankylosing spondylitis. If the examiner asks you:

E – *Where else would you like to examine?*

Other systems affected could be: lungs (expansion and apical fibrosis); heart (aortic incompetence); eyes (acute iritis)

It is unlikely that the exam would include a patient with root irritation because of the pain. However, the examiner may extend the station by:

E – *If you found that the patient had limited straight leg raising, weak dorsiflexion of the left foot and loss of ankle jerk, what conclusions would you draw?*
S – *I think that the most likely diagnosis would be an L5 root lesion, possibly due to disc prolapse.*
E *What would you do next?*

The first investigation would be a plain radiograph looking for joint space loss and vertebral disease. The best imaging technique is magnetic resonance. You might also suggest systemic investigations such as an ESR (e.g. myeloma).

EXAMINATION 21 Shoulder examination

Level:	**
Setting:	Normal volunteer
Time:	5 min

TASK

E – *Please show me how you would examine the shoulder of this patient.*

RESPONSE

It is unlikely that patients will be included in the examination, most likely you will be asked to examine a normal shoulder. The most common, stable, shoulder problem would be a frozen shoulder in which the movement would be very restricted.

Core skill: Examination of the shoulder

1. Observation:
   - Wasting.

2. Palpation:
   - Tenderness
   - Swelling
   - Crepitus on movement.

3. Movement:
   - Abduction
   - Adduction
   - Flexion
   - Extension
   - Internal rotation.

The shoulder is a complicated joint that is held in a place by the surrounding muscles and ligaments. It has a wide range of movement, which is further extended by the movement of the scapula on the posterior chest wall.

Observation

The joint is covered by the deltoid muscle and is surrounded by the rotator cuff muscles. The deltoid, in particular, may waste in any proximal myopathy. Effusions in the shoulder are usually not visible unless very large.

Palpation

Feel (and *comment on*) any pain or swelling (bogginess) of the joint as well as crepitus on movement.

Movement

The starting position should be the arm hanging by the side of the body with the palm facing the body. You should examine movement by standing behind the patient. For the right shoulder, use your left hand to overlap the scapula and superior part of the shoulder muscle. This allows you to fix the scapula and detect whether apparent movement of the shoulder is mainly due to the scapula sliding on the chest wall. Use your right hand to move the arm in the way described below. During all the movements, you should comment on limitation with and without pain and joint crepitus.

Abduction
Grip the elbow and *abduct* the arm. This initial movement is at the glenohumeral joint and usually can occur to 90°. The palm is then rotated anteriorly and can be further abducted to around 180°.

Adduction
Move the arm across the front of the chest. Normally, the shoulder can adduct to 50°.

External rotation
Ask the person to bend the elbow to 90°. Rotate the arm laterally as far as possible (normal up to 60°).

Internal rotation
Turn the arm in towards the chest wall (normal 90°).

Flexion
Elevate and move the arm forward as far as possible (180°).

Extension
With the elbow bent to 90°, move the arm backwards (65°).

Mostly, disease within the joint (intra-articular) causes painful movement in all directions, whereas tendonitis produces pain in one plane of movement (e.g. the painful arc on initial abduction with supraspinatus tendonitis). Neurological lesions or tendon rupture results in painless weakness.

SUGGESTIONS FOR FURTHER PRACTICE

Either orthopaedic or rheumatology clinics are the only places in which you will commonly see patients with shoulder problems. You should practise the examination on the patients that you examine for other reasons. You can also use your fellow students.

Extension to station (Level: ***)

It would be difficult to find sufficient patients with similar shoulder joint problems for a large scale OSCE. The most common is probably a frozen shoulder, in which movement is limited in all planes. The station could be extended by showing you a radiograph with degenerative changes.

EXAMINATION 22 — Examine the hands

Level:	**
Setting:	A patient with hand deformity (rheumatoid arthritis)
Time:	5 min

TASK

E – *Please examine this patient's hands. During your examination, I want you to tell me what you are doing and what you find.*

S – *Do you want me to examine the peripheral nervous system?*

E – *Confine yourself to the joints.*

RESPONSE

All joint examination can be divided into three stages:

1. General inspection
2. Examine the joint affected
3. Look for, and examine, other joints that are involved.

For individual joints the same steps are used:

- Inspection – deformity, swelling, skin changes, muscle wasting
- Palpation – swelling, tenderness, local heat, effusion
- Range of movement – active/passive
- Joint stability.

Core skill: Joint examination of hands

1. Ask whether the patient's hands are painful before touching them.

2. Inspect both the palm and dorsum of the hands and comment on the presence of any deformity, swelling and other abnormalities.

3. Palpate individual joints and comment on any tenderness or localised swelling.

4. Examine mobility/movement and comment on any limitation of movement or pain on movement of individual joints.

5. Assess grip and pinch strength.

At the end of the examination the examiner asks:

E – *What is your diagnosis and where else would you look to confirm this?*

EXAMINATION SKILLS

147

In this station, the patient has rheumatoid arthritis, so applying the system set out above:

Inspection

- Look for muscle wasting of the intrinsic muscles.
- Comment on any ulnar (common) or radial (rare) deviation.
- In the fingers, look for *swan neck* or *boutonnière* deformities.
- Examine the nails for any vasculitic changes.
- Comment on any evidence of surgery suggesting joint replacement or tendon repair.

Palpation

- Palpate each of the joints in turn: wrist, metacarpals, PIPs and DIPS. At each set of joints, comment on synovitis and deformity.
- For the diagnosis of rheumatoid disease, you should check for symmetry of the arthropathy and sparing of the DIPs. There may be tenderness over the ulnar styloid.

Range of movements

- Demonstrate the active/passive range of each joint (set of joints).
- Examine the function of the hand – patients can use hands that are very deformed. Test the patient's hand and pinch grip strength. You can also request them to undo a button or write.
- There may be crepitus over the tendon sheaths when extending/flexing the fingers.

Joint stability

- Comment on any subluxation of joints (see deformities above) and arthritis mutulans (more common in psoriatic arthropathy).

Look elsewhere

- In particular, ask to examine over the elbows and extensor surfaces of the forearms for rheumatoid nodules.

SUGGESTIONS FOR FURTHER PRACTICE

The best place to see patients with arthritic changes is in the rheumatology clinic. Most patients with active arthropathy are no longer admitted to hospital.

EXAMINATION SKILLS

Extensions to station (Levels: **/***)

The commonest cause of hand deformity due to arthritis is osteoarthritis. In this, the main features are:

- The DIPs are the commonest joints affected.
- The 1st carpo-metacarpal joint ('squaring') is also frequently affected.
- Heberden's nodes at the DIPs and Bouchard's nodes at the PIPs.

More rarely, you will encounter patients with psoriatic arthritis. In this, the examiner will want you to comment on:

- The nail changes (pitting, ridging, onycholysis – nail bed separation).
- The severity of the deformity ('arthritis mutilans').
- The asymmetry of the arthritis.

EXAMINATION 23   # Examine the hip

Level:	**
Setting:	Examine a patient with a hip problem
Time:	10 min

TASK

E – *Please show me how you would examine this patient's hips.*

RESPONSE

A patient with a hip problem in an OSCE most likely has osteoarthrosis. This is going to lead to some restriction (and possible pain) on movement – if you observe this when the patient is getting onto the couch (or during the examination) you should comment on it.

Core skill: Hip examination

A basic check list for examination of the hip is:

1. Comment on any restriction or pain on movement.

2. Comment on any swelling/skin discolouration over the hip.

3. Comment on any tenderness over the joint (and allow for it in your examination).

4. Ask the patient to move the joint through: flexion, rotation, abduction, adduction and extension and estimate any restriction in movement.

5. Passively move the joint through the same movement and look for differences compared to the active movements.

6. Measure true leg length.

7. Finally, ask the patient to walk and observe the gait.

After you have completed your examination, the second part of the station may develop in this way:

E – *So how would you interpret your findings?*
S – *Given this patient's age, the limitation of rotation and abduction to about 25°, I would think that the most likely diagnosis is osteoarthrosis.*
E – *So what investigation would you like to do?*
S – *Er ... some basic blood tests.*
E – *They are unlikely to be of much help, the ESR may be mildly increased if there is*

some inflammation and the haemoglobin reduced if the patient has been taking NSAIDs and has been losing blood. What is the best investigation?

S – *I suppose an X-ray.*

E – *Right, now look at this radiograph and tell me what you think.*

The student did well on the first part of the station, then started to become vague and would probably not have been able to justify the need for 'blood tests'. The examiner does not accept this general answer and tries to get to the point. Even then, the student does not sound definite and is probably worried about what comes next! However, the student is losing marks as the examiner's mark sheet probably includes:

- Ability to use appropriate investigations (radiographs)
- Ability to interpret radiographs.

In terms of general hip examination:

- *Observation* of the hip joint is not very useful as it is overlaid with muscle. You should comment on any muscle wasting, particularly of the quadriceps (hip flexor).
- *Palpation* – comment on any tenderness.
- *Movement* – have the patient lying on their back. Expose the legs, but make sure that the patient will not be exposed when you are testing abduction and adduction.
  - Flexion – flex the knee (so you are not doing a straight leg raise test), move the thigh towards the patient's chest. *Make sure that the pelvis does not rise from the bed.*
  - Rotation – Have the knee and hip flexed to about 90°. One hand holds the knee, the other foot. Move the foot medially (tests *external* rotation – normally about 45°). Move the foot laterally (*internal* rotation – 45°).
  - Abduction – grasp the heel of the leg with one hand, the other should fix the pelvis by pressing over the anterior superior iliac spine on the opposite side. Move the leg outwards as far as possible (50°).
  - Adduction – move the leg medially (45°).
  - Extension – have the patient turn over on to their stomach. Place one hand over the sacroiliac joint, the other hand elevates the leg (30°).
- Measure the leg length. The *true* length is measured from the anterior superior iliac crest on that side to the medial malleolus. The *apparent* length is from the umbilicus to the medial malleolus. A difference in true leg length (right compared to left) indicates hip disease on the shorter side. Apparent difference in leg length is due to tilting of the pelvis.

Include examination of gait in your assessment wherever it is relevant. This is likely to be so in neurological and rheumatological disease (see Table 4.3).

In osteoarthrosis, the early features will be restriction in rotation, abduction and adduction. There are no blood markers for osteoarthrosis. The most appropriate investigation is a plain radiograph which may show:

- osteophyte formation

- loss of joint space
- juxta-articular sclerosis
- bone cysts.

SUGGESTION FOR FURTHER PRACTICE

Observation of gait is an important part of examination (locomotor and neurological). You should make sure you can interpret the different gait patterns (Table 4.3). Has your library any suitable video collections?

Apart from knee examination, joint examination is a skill that most students lack confidence in. You need to seek out stable patients that you can practise on. In medicine, rheumatology clinics are the obvious source, but these may be over-subscribed by students or held infrequently in your hospital. You should also consider:

- Orthopaedic clinics – large, frequent clinics, mostly osteoarthrosis, but also some inflammatory arthropathies.
- Elderly care medicine – out-patients or rehabilitation units (ortho-geriatric units). Generally very good for patients with lots of physical signs, but patients less robust (for long practice sessions!).

EXAMINATION 24	**Examine the knee**
Level:	**/***
Setting:	Examine a patient with osteoarthritis
Time:	5 min

TASK

E – *The patient has some problem with the left knee. Please examine the knees.*

RESPONSE

As with the previous station, what the examiners are looking for is a thorough, systematic examination and your ability to detect and interpret physical signs. A crucial aspect is demonstrating awareness of any discomfort for the patient – this is very important in any similar station. Most mark sheets will contain criteria/ items relating to how you interact with the patient and how you show sensitivity to any distress. In locomotor problems, it is highly likely that the patient may experience discomfort either on palpation or on movement. If you anticipate this, it is easier to respond appropriately.

Core skill: Knee examination

1. Show awareness to any discomfort for the patient.

2. Expose and inspect both knees (thighs/calves).

3. Comment on any difference between the temperature of the knees.

4. Examine and comment on bony/synovial swelling.

5. Examine for, and comment on, the presence of effusions.

6. Demonstrate any differences in active and passive range of movements.

7. Demonstrate any lateral and AP stability.

In examination of the knee, the standard approach is:

Inspection

- Make sure that both knees are exposed, including the quadriceps muscle.
- Is there any swelling? If so, is it localised (suggesting a bursa, bony overgrowth) or generalised?
- Are there any skin changes – erythema, signs of suppuration (e.g. discharging fistula)?

153

- What is the position of the joint – is it in flexion or extension? Is there any deformity of position (*Genu varus* – 'knock knees', or *Genu valgus* – 'bow legs')?
- Is there any muscle wasting of the quadriceps?

Palpation

The patient should be in a relaxed position with the knees resting on the couch. Ask the patient if the joint hurts at all – if so then adjust your examination to take this into account. You should palpate for:

- Tenderness – is it localised to one spot or generalised?
- Swelling – is this generalised (effusion) or localised (synovium/bursa/bone)? Is it soft tissue or bone (hard)?
- Effusion:
  With a **large** effusion, the joint will be tense and grossly swollen with loss of landmarks. For a **small** effusion, you can use two manoeuvres to demonstrate the fluid:
  a. With one hand over the thigh just above the patella and pushing down the leg towards the foot, use the other hand to press down sharply on the patella and release. You are feeling a 'patella tap' meaning that the patella is 'floating' off the tibia/femur and can be tapped onto the bone.
  b. Stroke firmly with one hand over the medial bursa to empty it. Push over the lateral bursa and observe whether the medial border of the joint 'bulges' as the fluid is pushed back into the medial compartment.

Movement

Observe whether the knee is extended at rest, or, if flexed, estimate the angle with the lower limb (e.g. limb held at 15° flexion).

- Active movement: ask the patient to flex the joint as far as they can and estimate the degree of flexion. Observe/ask whether it is painful.
- Passive movement: move the joint through its range as far as you can without hurting the patient. Can it be extended fully? Can it be flexed to 160–170°?
- Palpate for any crepitus (cracking) from the joint as it is moved.

Stability

- AP stability (cruciate ligaments): ask the patient to place the sole of the foot on the bed so that the knee is flexed to around 90° and the quadriceps relaxed. Wrapping both hands around the joint so that your thumbs are over the anterior surface, 'draw' (pull) the leg towards you. Does the tibia 'move' towards you and away from the knee?
- Lateral stability (lateral ligaments): with the knee relaxed on the bed, fix the thigh with one hand. Place the other hand underneath the lower leg and move it gently from side to side. Is there an abnormal range of movement (should be minimal) indicating lateral ligament instability?

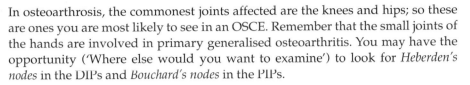

In osteoarthrosis, the commonest joints affected are the knees and hips; so these are ones you are most likely to see in an OSCE. Remember that the small joints of the hands are involved in primary generalised osteoarthritis. You may have the opportunity ('Where else would you want to examine') to look for *Heberden's nodes* in the DIP's and *Bouchard's nodes* in the PIP's.

This station involves a patient with knee osteoarthrosis. On examination, you may find that the joint is swollen due either to bony overgrowth or an effusion. It is likely that there will be limitation of movement, crepitus, deformity and instability. You should carefully demonstrate and comment on these. If you find that the joint is hot, this points to inflammation. One important complication to look for is a *Baker's cyst* in the knee, which consists of a degenerative out-pouching of the synovium which can be palpated in the popliteal fossa.

SUGGESTIONS FOR FURTHER PRACTICE

The easiest way to see patients with osteoarthrosis is in an orthopaedic clinic. Alternatively, you could try to see patients being admitted for joint replacement (who are likely to have gross changes).

Extension to station (Level: ***)

The easiest way to extend the station would be to ask 'what investigations would you do?' You should suggest a radiograph. This may show:

- Loss of joint space
- Osteophyte formation
- Sclerosis at the joint margins
- Bone cysts close to joint margins.

The examiner may also ask you to comment on a report of joint aspiration showing crystals of calcium pyrophosphate (weakly positive birefringent). These are seen in pseudogout (there may also be a faint line of calcification along the middle of the joint space on the radiograph).

EXAMINATION SKILLS

EXAMINATION 25	**Examine the skin**
Level:	✱✱✱
Setting:	Examine a patient with psoriasis, contact dermatitis or eczema
Time:	10–15 min

TASK

E – *Could you please talk to this patient and look at their skin condition. I want you to tell me what you think the problem is.*

RESPONSE

Dermatology is a very large branch of medicine, which is often not covered well in undergraduate curricula. Within OSCEs, there would be little point in using a normal volunteer at a station. It is easy for exam organisers to identify patients with psoriasis, dermatitis or eczema. The important aspect of dermatology is determining and recognising the overall pattern of skin involvement.

This station could be described as an OSLER (Objective Structured Long Examination Record) as it combines history, examination and differential diagnosis.

In the dermatological history, you should consider:

- When and where the rash began.
- Distribution.
- Any change over time.
- Relationship to sun exposure, heat or cold.
- Response to treatment.
- Is it itchy? *Localised* pruritus is usually due to dermatological problems.
- Is there any pain or disturbed sensation?
- Are there any constitutional symptoms such as weight loss, fatigue, headache?

In the past medical history, you should ask about:

- Previous rashes or allergic reactions.
- Atopy as suggested by a previous asthma, eczema or hay fever.
- Any systemic disease – e.g. diabetes or inflammatory bowel disease.

In the social history:

- Occupation
- Hobbies
- Chemical exposure or contact with animals or plants
- What tablets the patient is taking (very common cause of skin problems in a general medical patient).

Family history

- Atopy, other members of family affected (remember skin infestation through close contact).

When you move on to your examination, you should have some idea of what the problem is likely to be and you then confirm (or not) your impression. In a thorough dermatological examination, the patient should be undressed and the whole skin surface and appendages carefully inspected. In a short OSCE station, this may not be possible, but you should indicate that this is what you would do.

Core skill: Skin examination

1. Take a careful history including:
   - Past medical history
   - Allergies
   - Atopy
   - Systemic disease
   - Occupation
   - Hobbies
   - Medication
   - Family history.

2. Expose the skin as much as possible.

3. Generalised skin problem?

4. Distribution and type of rash/abnormality:
   - Solid, red, non-scaling
   - Solid, red, scaling
   - Solid, not red
   - Fluid-filled.

In this station, you must be able to recognise: psoriasis, eczema and contact or allergic dermatitis.

Comment on (by inspection and palpation):

- Is there a general skin problem such as widespread excoriation suggesting intense generalised pruritus?
- Is any rash generalised or localised? If the latter, what is the distribution?
- Is the rash:
  - *Solid, red, non-scaling* (e.g. erythema nodosum, erythema multiforme)?
  - *Solid, red, scaling?*
    - ♦ If the epithelium is disrupted then consider atopic dermatitis or contact dermatitis (look at the pattern)
    - ♦ If the epithelium is intact consider psoriasis

- *Solid, not red*
    - ♦ Skin coloured – warts, skin cancer, sebacious cyst
    - ♦ White patch, e.g. vitiligo or papules, e.g. molluscum contagiosum
    - ♦ Brown/black patch, e.g. café au lait lesions or nodules/papules, e.g. melanoma, naevus
    - *Fluid-filled* – if clear vesicles, consider conditions such as herpes zoster, pemphigoid. If pustular, consider acne vulgaris or infection.

In this station, the main conditions would be:

Psoriasis

Scaly, red lesions with well demarcated edge, usually over extensor surfaces. Also look for any nail changes (pitting, onycholysis).

Eczema

Atopic eczema is usually in the skin flexures with erythema and fine scaling. It may become chronic with cracking and secondary infection. There are also other varieties such as nummular eczema, which causes widespread diffuse coin lesions that are intensely pruritic.

Contact or allergic dermatitis

Any potent skin irritant can cause localised inflammation with erythema, scaling and cracking. Differentiating dermatitis from eczema can be difficult, particularly when it is confined to the hands. A detailed history is very important.

SUGGESTIONS FOR FURTHER PRACTICE

Diagnosis in dermatology is principally about pattern recognition. The more you have seen the variety of ways in which psoriasis can present, the more confident you will be in making the diagnosis. You should take any opportunity to go to dermatology clinics. There are also CAL packages and colour atlases that beautifully illustrate the spectrum of skin disorders.

Extension to station (Level: ***)

The station could easily be extended by showing you pictures of other common skin problems and asking you to describe the abnormality and what the likely diagnosis is. In an OSLER, the examiners could ask you for your initial management (e.g. stop exposure in contact dermatitis, simple emollients such as E45 cream and oilatum, increasing potency of steroids for eczema and allergic dermatitis).

CHAPTER 5

DATA INTERPRETATION

Introduction

Stations involving data are very common in OSCEs because they are easy to set up and do not require volunteers, patients, standardised patients or specialised pieces of equipment (apart from a viewing box for radiographs). The most common form is a structured viva with an examiner who:

- Gives you some information (clinical description, images, data, ECG, radiographs, biopsies) and asks for your interpretation.
- Asks you what you would do next.
- Gives you more information to link in.

You do not have to get the first bit correct to move onto the second stage. Nor do you have to suggest the next correct investigation. The examiner will steer you there to see how you get on with some more information. What the examiner is interested in is how you work through a problem as more data are added.

Sometimes, the station will not have an examiner present. You will be required to interpret the information presented as a package and write a response (this could be in the form of a referral letter to a specialist or an entry into a patient's case-notes). These stations are little different from a classical OSCE format, but allow expansion of the number of OSCE stations at minimum cost and effort.

Examiners will expect you to know the normal ranges for the common tests such as urea and electrolytes, blood glucose and full blood count. For other, less commonplace investigations, the reference range is likely to be given alongside the results. We have provided tables of reference ranges at the end of the book.

This section gives some examples of data stations. You will find many more questions of a type that you may well find in OSCE stations in the Medicine book of the Master of Medicine series, published by Harcourt Publishers.

DATA 1 — Urea and electrolytes

Level:	*
Setting:	Structured oral
Time:	10 min

TASK

E – *You are looking through the biochemical results from the patients you are currently looking after. You come across this report of a 70-year-old woman. What is your interpretation of the results?*

> Biochemistry
>
> | | |
> |---|---|
> | Urea | 19.6 mmol/l |
> | Creatinine | 192 µmol/l |
> | Sodium | 135 mmol/l |
> | Potassium | 3.0 mmol/l |
> | Chloride | 100 mmol/l |
> | Bicarbonate | 25 mmol/l |

E – *What do you think is the most likely cause in this patient?*

RESPONSE

A basic skill is interpretation of urea and electrolyte results. In this case, the patient has a raised urea and creatinine and a low potassium. The most likely cause is over-treatment with a diuretic, but a low potassium can be due to steroid (prednisolone) therapy.

E – *The patient was known to have stable heart failure with controlled atrial fibrillation. She had had the blood test because she had lost her appetite and was feeling sick. She was also feeling dizzy when she got up in the morning. What do you think are the causes of the patient's symptoms?*

The patient's symptoms are consistent with over-diuresis causing postural hypotension. It is also likely that the patient is on digoxin to control their ventricular response to the atrial fibrillation. The worsening renal function would cause a reduction in the digoxin excretion and subsequent toxicity.

E – *What would you look for on examination? The patient is on 80 mg of frusemide and 0.1875 mg of digoxin; what would you do next?*

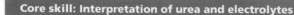

> **Core skill: Interpretation of urea and electrolytes**
>
> 1. Check patient details:
>   - Gender, date of birth (renal function deteriorates with age – loss of approx 1 ml GFR per year)
>
> 2. Check basic indices:
>   - Urea
>   - Creatinine
>   - Sodium
>   - Potassium
>   - Chloride
>   - Bicarbonate.
>
> 3. If raised urea and creatinine – suggests renal impairment. Should discuss measurement of renal function (creatinine clearance), and whether pre-renal, renal or post-renal failure.
>
> 4. If urea elevated, but creatinine not to same degree – suggests GI bleed with 'protein meal' or reduced renal blood flow due to volume depletion/diuretic therapy (for CCF).
>
> 5. If urea low – unusual, can be seen in liver failure.
>
> 6. High potassium – most common in renal failure.
>
> 7. Low potassium – most commonly due to diuretics.
>
> 8. High sodium – most commonly due to water depletion (not taking fluids).
>
> 9. Low sodium – most commonly due to drugs (carbamazepine) – inappropriate ADH secretion or i.v. dextrose post-surgery.
>
> 10. Bicarbonate – indicates alkalosis (high) or acidosis (low).

You should direct your examination to the probable volume depletion with digoxin toxicity. You will need to perform a careful cardiovascular examination, including pulse rate (apex, radial) and postural blood pressure. Look at Procedure 8: Venous cannulation for discussion of how to assess volume depletion and choose an appropriate replacement fluid.

The management must include stopping digoxin temporarily, reducing the diuretic dose and prescribing potassium supplements. The patient may benefit from an ACE inhibitor or a potassium sparing diuretic (amiloride, triamterine) in the longer term.

SUGGESTION FOR FURTHER PRACTICE

You should be able to discuss the common abnormalities seen in urea and

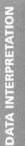

electrolyte results (including symptoms and signs, further investigation and initial management):

- Low/high sodium
- Low/high potassium
- High urea and creatinine.

You should also revise:

- Low/high calcium.

DATA 2	**Chest radiograph**
Level:	**
Setting:	Structured oral with examiner, material provided
Time:	10 min

TASK

E – *In your ward is a 48-year-old man who has been admitted with weight loss and general malaise. He is a heavy smoker and drinks quite a lot. He has been living in bed and breakfast accommodation. On examination, his temperature is 37.4°C, he looks cachexic. There is nothing else to find on examination. How would you proceed?*

RESPONSE

In this patient, the presentation is quite vague with no pointers to any system. It is likely that the examiner will steer you towards discussing his way of life. Smoking always raises the possibility of bronchial carcinoma, heavy drinking links to liver disease, but also poor nutrition. People who live permanently in bed and breakfast accommodation often do not look after themselves very well. Tuberculosis must be a strong possibility in view of these factors.

The principal clue for the next stage of investigation is the pyrexia suggesting infection. This could be secondary to bronchial obstruction behind a tumour or could be related to airflow obstruction. A chest radiograph is required, but you could also justify:

- Full blood count – raised white cell count, but also macrocytosis due to alcohol
- Liver function tests – alcohol, evidence of malnutrition (albumen)
- Blood cultures – pyrexia
- Mid-stream urine – bacterial infection, also sterile pyuria (TB)
- Sputum sample (if possible) – Gram stain, culture and ZN stain/culture.

E – *I would like you to look at this chest radiograph (Fig. 5.1) and tell me what you think.*

The most important core skill is your ability to interpret a chest radiograph. These are very common in OSCEs. It may show abnormalities of (or in combination):

- Lung/airway
- Heart
- Soft tissue
- Skeleton.

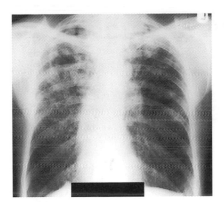

Figure 5.1 Chest radiograph

The key steps are shown in the box. In the film presented, the main abnormalities are apical shadowing with cavitation. These are principally in the right upper zone, but are also present on the left side. There may also be some distortion of the left hilum. This combination of *bilateral* apical shadowing with cavitation is

Core skill: Interpretation of a chest radiograph

1. Start off by checking name, date and orientation of the film.

2. State if it is an AP film (marked as such – causes apparent cardiomegaly), otherwise assume PA.

3. Describe any obvious abnormality in the lung fields or heart shape:
   - Use upper, mid and lower zone to describe site of any problem
   - Need lateral film to localise to lobes (because of the direction of the fissures).

4. If there are no abnormalities (and at the end) check and comment on:
   - Any problems behind the heart (need a penetrated film)
   - Any bulkiness at the hila (lymph nodes, tumour, vascular – pulmonary hypertension)
   - Retrosternal goitre
   - Presence of both breast shadows in a female patient
   - Skeleton (ribs, humerus, clavicle)
   - Soft tissues.

5. Lungs:
   - Upper lobe collapse causes tracheal deviation
   - Lower lobe collapse causes mediastinal shift and the left lobe collapses as a triangle behind the heart
   - The middle lobe collapses as a triangle adjacent to the right heart with loss of the border.

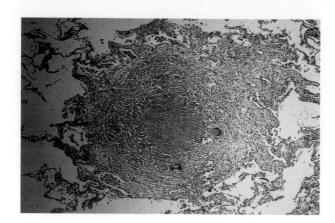

Figure 5.2

strongly suggested of TB. The hilar distortion points to previous damage with upper lobe fibrosis and traction on the hilar vessels.

E – *On the basis of your intepretation of the radiograph, what would you do now?*

The next stage would be to prove the tentative diagnosis. Mantoux testing would confirm previous exposure (always start at 1:10 000 dilution of tuberculin). A strong reaction (which may include skin ulceration at low dilution) is highly suggestive of active TB. However, this still falls short of proof. You need to confirm the presence of the bacillus. ZN stain and culture of sputum may be feasible, but many patients are not expectorating.

E – *The patient eventually had a bronchoscopy and a biopsy was taken (Fig. 5.2). Please describe this to me and what would you do now?*

A bronchoscopy with bronchial lavage is often very helpful. Direct biopsy is not usually carried out unless there are endobronchial lesions (rare). In miliary TB, a trans-bronchial biopsy can be diagnostic.

It is very easy to become anxious if shown a histopathology slide. It is likely that by this stage, you will have a clear idea of what the problem is (e.g. TB) and can then look for features on the slide that you know to be present in the particular condition.

Here, the biopsy shows a typical tuberculous granuloma with central caseation, surrounded by an inflammatory response with a few giant cells of Langerhans.

If you are shown a slide to start a station, you need to first identify the tissue that it has come from. Are there any clues from what the examiner has told you (e.g. this 37-year-old man has severe hypertension)? If you know that you are looking at kidney, it makes it much easier to consider what pathological process might be affecting that organ (e.g. glomerulonephritis). If you cannot identify the tissue, inform the examiner. You may not get the first mark, but it will save you time if

they tell you that it is liver you are looking at. You can then concentrate on whether it might be cirrhosis.

The other, more common approach, is to show you a pathology report with the diagnosis removed. In this case, there may be particular phrases that point to a diagnosis (e.g. Reed–Sternberg cells in Hodgkin's lymphoma).

In this station, having established the diagnosis, the next steps are:

- Notify the disease to the Public Health Department.
- Initiate treatment (triple therapy with isoniazid, rifampacin, pyrazinamide).
- Seek help from a consultant in respiratory medicine.

SUGGESTIONS FOR FURTHER PRACTICE

This station is typical of a structured oral in taking you from your initial clinical hypotheses, through the interpretation of a chest radiograph, your plan of investigation and finally the interpretation of a histopathology slide. Remember that there are marks for all the steps so do not panic if you get stuck, tell the examiner, who will almost certainly move on.

In preparation for the OSCE, you should:

- Go down to the Department of Radiology. There are often weekly displays and all departments have libraries of 'classic' films.
- Use the library for access to CAL packages on interpretation of radiographs and histopathology slides.
- On the worldwide web, there are very good teaching sites for radiology and histopathology – ask the librarian.
- Use the assessment sections of the Mastery of Medicine book. These have many questions linking data interpretation to clinical findings.

DATA INTERPRETATION

DATA 3	**Urinalyis**
Level:	**
Setting:	Structured oral with examiner, picture provided
Time:	10 min

TASK

E – *A 25-year-old man has been admitted under your care with increasing swelling of the face, hands and legs. He has also noticed some blurring of vision with headaches. The nurse who admitted him has tested the small amount of urine that he has passed.*

> Urine testing:
>
> John Wainwright
>
> pH: 6.2
> Glucose: negative
> Ketones: negative
> Nitrites: negative
> Protein: +++
> Red cells: +++
> White cells: ++

E – *What is the relevance of the urine test results?*

RESPONSE

The interpretation of basic urinary investigations is an important skill for house officers. You need to be able to recognise a number of basic patterns and initiate appropriate further assessment and investigations:

- Infection
- Proteinuria
- Haematuria
- Glomerular/renal tubular disease.

A scheme for interpretation is shown in the box.

In this patient, there are significant amounts of protein and red and white cells. This might imply infection, but the test for nitrites is negative. The other alternative is renal disease (glomerular or tubular). This is strongly supported by the widespread oedema, which suggests either acute nephritis or nephrotic syndrome.

Core skill: Interpretation of urine tests

Urine is usually screened using a strip test allowing multiple analysis of pH, glucose, ketones, blood, nitrite, specific gravity, presence of leucocytes, bile and urobilinogen.

1. pH: if urine is alkaline suspect either *Proteus mirabilis* infection (splits urea) or distal renal tubular acidosis.

2. Protein: anything greater than '+' is abnormal – if present, you should do a 24-h excretion measurement. If a '+' persists and is not due to infection – 24-h measurement.

3. Glycosuria suggests (the strips are oversensitive) diabetes mellitus (remember low renal threshold in pregnancy).

4. Ketones suggest diabetic ketoacidosis or starvation (e.g. after surgery).

5. Nitrites: presence indicates infection.

6. White cells: indicate infection or renal disease (sterile pyuria in renal TB).

7. Red cells: microscopic haematuria should be investigated – renal disease, carcinoma.

E – *In your examination, the fundal appearances are shown below. What would you do immediately?*

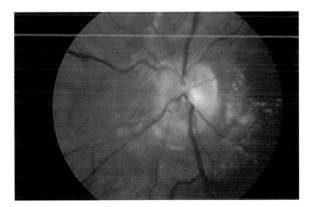

Figure 5.3

Eye examination including fundoscopy is discussed in Examination 10. Here, the picture shows grade IV hypertensive retinopathy with papilloedema. Given that nephrotic syndrome causes hypovolaemia due to loss of protein, the diagnosis must be acute nephritis. This is a medical emergency and you should contact the senior members of your team, measure the urea and electrolytes and get in touch with the nearest renal centre. The patient is at risk of fitting or intra-cerebral haemorrhage due to high blood pressure. The immediate management is to put the patient on strict bed-rest and reduce the diastolic BP to no lower than 100 mmHg in 12–24 h. Various drug treatments are used, for example sub-lingual nifedipine combined with an oral beta-blocker.

E – *You have gone on to ask for urine microscopy and culture amongst other investigations and immediate management. How do you interpret the results?*

> John Wainwright:
>
> Urine: no growth
> Red cells: 80/lpf
> White cells: 20/lpf
> Red cells: predominantly dysmorphic
> Numerous red cell casts

In addition to diagnosing urinary infection, microscopy can be very useful in possible renal disease.

- Red blood cells: usually none, but may be up to 5/low powered field (lpf). If the cells originate from the glomeruli rather than the renal tract, then a high percentage will be dysmorphic (irregular in size and shape).
- White blood cells: usually fewer than 6/lpf. Pyuria indicates urinary tract inflammation.
- Casts are cylindrical shapes formed in the lumen of the tubules or collecting ducts:
  - Hyaline: renal tubules. Tamm–Horsfall mucoprotein with very few cells
  - Granular: usually tubules
  - Red cell: always abnormal and indicate primary glomerular disease.

In this station, the microscopy is consistent with glomerular disease.

SUGGESTIONS FOR FURTHER PRACTICE

This station combines renal disease, hypertension and eye problems. You will improve your understanding of them (and the related skills) by visiting:

- Dialysis unit, renal clinics
- Hypertension clinics
- Ophthalmology units.

DATA INTERPRETATION

DATA 4	**Cerebrospinal fluid**
Level:	*
Setting:	Structured oral with examiner, data provided
Time:	10 min

TASK

E – *You see a patient in Casualty. He is a 27-year-old man who started with back pain 8 days ago. He then noticed pins and needles in his feet and increasing difficulty in walking. What would you look for on examination?*

RESPONSE

This station links in with Examinations 14 and 16 (neurological examination of legs). The initial step is to distinguish between a peripheral and a central nervous system lesion. The back pain points towards the spinal cord and the main differential diagnoses are:

- Cord compression
- Guillain–Barré syndrome
- Multiple sclerosis (less likely with back pain).

You should tell the examiner that you would perform a careful neurological examination looking for:

- Evidence of upper motor neurone signs (points towards cord compression above L1/L2 verterbra)
- Sensory level
- Full bladder and lax anal tone (autonomic dysfunction due to cord compression – neuro-surgical emergency. In Guillain–Barré, autonomic disturbance is only seen in very severe cases).

You might also suggest baseline pulmonary function tests (e.g. peak flow rate) in view of the possible Guillain–Barré syndrome.

E – *On examination, you find that he is apyrexial. There is no spinal tenderness. You cannot elicit any reflexes in his legs and power is reduced particularly distally. He has disturbed sensation from T12 downwards with complete loss below his knees. His bladder is not palpable and anal tone is normal. What would you do next?*

The initial presentation with back pain and then ascending paralysis and sensory disturbance is typical of Guillain–Barré syndrome. However, if there is any possibility of cord compression, you should request plain spinal radiographs and then magnetic resonance imaging, which must be done as an emergency.

Delay in diagnosing and treating cord compression significantly reduces the chances of good recovery.

Examination of the cerebrospinal fluid is very helpful in confirming Guillain–Barré syndrome.

E – *The CSF findings from the lumbar puncture are shown below.*
How do you interpret these findings?

Red cell count/high powered field	5
White cell count/high powered field	7
Protein g/l	1.3
CSF glucose mmol/l	3.8
Blood glucose mmol/l	4.9

The core skill in this station is interpretation of CSF results; the most common neurology dataset in OSCE (or other examinations). An approach is shown in the box and the specific changes are given in Table 5.1.

Core skill: Interpretation of CSF results

1. The key step is to establish the pattern of changes.

2. Look through the results and mark each of them as being very low, low, normal, high or very high.

3. State these to the examiners (e.g. *'the protein is normal'*) so that you can be given credit for the initial analysis.

4. Put these changes together as a pattern (e.g. raised cells, neutrophils, very low sugar, raised protein = probable bacterial meningitis).

5. Particular patterns can be due to a number of conditions (raised cells, lymphocytes, low sugar, normal/slight elevation of protein = viral meningitis, encephalitis etc. [see Table 5.1]).

6. For these patterns, look at what other information you have on the clinical presentation (e.g. bizarre behaviour would point towards encephalitis).

In this patient, the CSF initially shows a small increase in white cells, then, after about a week, the protein increases. However, cord compression can also cause a very high CSF protein level. You can confirm the diagnosis of Guillain–Barré with nerve conduction studies, which will show severe slowing of nerve conduction due to a demyelinating radiculopathy.

Table 5.1 Patterns of CSF abnormalities

	Pressure	Cells	Glucose	Protein
Bacterial meningitis	→ or ↑	↑ neut.	↓↓ or undect.	↑ or ↑↑
Viral meningitis		↑ lymph. early neut.	↓	Normal or slight ↑
Viral encephalitis		Mild ↑ lymph	↓	Normal or slight ↑
Brain abscess/ parameningeal focus	May ↑	↑ neut.	Normal or ↓	↑
Fungal meningitis	May ↑	↑ lymph	Normal or ↓	Normal or ↑
Tuberculous meningitis	May ↑	↑ lymph	↓↓	↑ or ↑↑
Malignancy		Malign.	↓	Some ↑
Guillain–Barré syndrome		Slight ↑	Normal	↑ after 1st week
Multiple sclerosis		Slight ↑ lymph	Normal	Mild ↑
Spinal cord compression			Normal	↑↑
Subarachnoid haemorrhage	May ↑	Red cell ↑↑	Normal	↑

SUGGESTIONS FOR FURTHER PRACTICE

Lumbar punctures are carried out almost daily on neurology wards. If you have never seen one, ask the nursing staff or junior doctor on the neurology ward in your hospital to let you know when one is due to be performed. Read communication 7: (lumbar puncture), for a description of the procedure and what it entails for the patient.

DATA INTERPRETATION

DATA 5	**Blood count**
Level:	**
Setting:	**Structured oral with examiner**
Time:	**10 min**

TASK

E – *A 72-year-old woman has been admitted onto the Programmed-Investigation Unit. The Unit sister has asked you to come to see the patient before she goes home to explain the results of her tests. The patient was admitted for tests because of the result of her full blood count.*

Full blood count

Haemoglobin	67 g/l
WCC	5.5
Platelets	220
PCV	0.29
MCV	66 fl
MCH	20 pg
MCHC	24

E – *What abnormalities are present and what is your diagnosis?*

RESPONSE

The patient has an iron deficiency anaemia as judged by the low haemoglobin, packed cell volume, mean cell volume (haematocrit) and mean cell haemoglobin concentration. The steps in the core skill of interpreting a full blood count are shown in the core skill box.

E – *What might you have asked the patient about and looked for on examination?*

Having established the diagnosis, the next step is to identify the cause. Most likely, this will be due to gastrointestinal blood loss. In a younger woman you would consider excessive menstrual blood loss. In this patient, you would ask directly about gastrointestinal symptoms and use of non-steroidal anti-inflammatory drugs. You should tell the examiner that you would perform a general physical examination, a thorough abdominal examination and a rectal examination.

E – *What tests would you have ordered?*

The next stage is to confirm the diagnosis through estimation of serum ferritin

Core skill: Interpretation of full blood count

1. Look at the patient details:
   - Male/female and date of birth (age), which make a difference in the differential diagnosis (e.g. menstrual blood loss).

2. Check that the basic indices are normal:
   - Hb
   - WCC
   - Platelets.

3. If raised or low, is this a minimal or a gross change? Try to establish any links between the abnormalities (e.g. elevation of all three would suggest polycythaemia rubra vera).

4. Check the ESR – is this elevated (e.g. myeloma or giant cell arteritis)?

5. Look at the red cell indices:
   - Microcytosis/macrocytosis
   - Low mean cell haemoglobin concentration (iron deficiency)
   - Raised packed cell volume (erythrocytosis).

6. Look at the white cell count differential indices:
   - Is there a neutrophilia or neutropenia?
   - Is there a lymphocytosis or lymphopenia?

(but is increased in inflammation – acute phase reactant) or serum iron and iron-binding capacity. You should state that it would be wrong to simply put the patient on iron. Faecal occult bloods are of no help in this situation, you must image the gastrointestinal tract through barium studies and/or endoscopy.

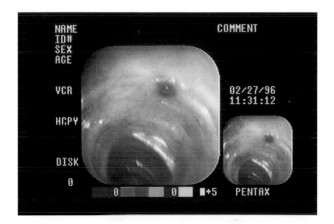

Figure 5.4

E – *A colonoscopy was carried out and a report and a picture has been sent back to the unit. Many of the abnormalities on the picture were seen. What abnormality has been identified on the colonoscopy? What would you tell the patient?*

In this case, the colonoscopy has not shown a polyp or colonic carcinoma as the usual cause of blood loss. The small raised areas are due to angiodysplasia, which is a common cause of iron deficiency anaemia in elderly people, particularly when a barium enema is negative. Given this information, you need to consider how you would discuss the findings with the patient (see Communication 13: Give information to a patient).

SUGGESTIONS FOR FURTHER PRACTICE

You should be able to recognise the FBC patterns commonly used in OSCEs stations:

- Fe deficiency
- Megaloblastic anaemia
- Polycythaemia rubra vera
- Secondary erythrocytosis
- Leukaemia
- Aplastic anaemia.

DATA INTERPRETATION

DATA 6	**Deliberate self-harm**
Level:	**
Setting:	Structured oral with examiner
Time:	5–10 min

TASK

E – *You are the house officer on call for medicine and are asked to see a 23-year-old woman in a distressed state, who has been brought to Casualty by a paramedical crew and is saying that she has taken 'a lot of tablets'. What would you do?*

RESPONSE

As a house officer, you are going to see a lot of patients with deliberate self-harm. It follows that OSCEs (and other assessments) are likely to include such problems. For any patient with possible poisoning, the core skill in assessment is shown in the box.

Core skill: Assessment of deliberate self-harm

1. Assessment of airways, breathing and cardiac ('ABC') followed by conscious level (Glasgow coma scale see Table 5.2).

2. Ascertain what the patient has taken *and obtain independent confirmation if possible* (see bottles, talk to paramedics, friends etc.).

3. Make assessment (history and examination) of possible toxicity (e.g. tachycardia, hypotension, tremor etc.).

4. Organise appropriate initial investigations.

5. Give supportive treatment (e.g. fluid, oxygen) and any specific treatment/antidotes that are indicated.

6. Make assessment of psychological state and possible suicidal risk.

7. Continue to monitor for improvement/deterioration.

E – *You find out that she has taken only aspirin.*
Can you give some investigations you would do and why?

For this patient, appropriate initial investigations would be salicylate levels, urea and electrolytes, blood gases and blood glucose. Others might include urine pH, chest radiograph (pulmonary oedema in late stages), prothrombin time (hypoprothrombinaemia) and ECG (hypokalaemia).

DATA INTERPRETATION

Table 5.2 Glasgow coma scale

Category		Score
Eye opening		
Spontaneous		4
To speech		3
To pain		2
None		1
Best verbal response (needs 6)		
Orientated		5
Confused		4
Inappropriate		3
Incomprehensible		2
None		1
Best motor response:		
To verbal command	Obeys	6
To painful stimui	Localising	5
Flexion	Withdrawal	4
Flexion (Decorticate rigidity)	Abnormal	3
Extension (Decerebrate rigidity)		2
None		1

In any station which has a scenario of a patient with a reduced level of consciousness, the examiner would **expect** you to know the Glasgow coma scale and may ask you to calculate it for the described case.
Note: The scores are summed to give an overall rating between 3 and 15; minimum score is 3.

E – *Here are the results of some investigations:*

Salicylates	821 mg/l
Urea	4.5 mmo/l
Sodium	135 mmol/l
Potassium	3.0 mmol/l
Blood gases	
pH	7.2
PaO_2	13.6 kPa
$PaCO_2$	3.3 kPa
HCO_3	14 mmol/l

E – *How do you explain these results and what other features might you look for confirming severe poisoning by salicylates?*

The results show high salicylate levels, hypokalaemia and metabolic acidosis with respiratory alkalosis, consistent with severe toxicity. See Procedure 15 for discussion of arterial blood sampling and interpretation of results.

Confirmatory features of severe salicylate toxicity include :

1. Fever, sweating (due to uncoupling oxidative phosphorylation)
2. Confusion (neuroglycopenia)
3. Epigastric discomfort, vomiting (delayed gastric emptying)
4. Tachypnoea (in adults, direct stimulation resp. centre)
5. Pre-renal failure (volume depletion)
6. Hypo- or hyperglycaemia, hypo- or hypernatraemia
7. Pulmonary oedema (late feature).

It is important to know that severely poisoned patients may not lose consciousness until just prior to death.

E – *What would be your management?*

In terms of management, you need to stratify the degree of toxicity into three grades (levels given are 6-h post-poisoning):

1. Mild poisoning (< 500 mg/l) – fluid and electrolyte balance alone (i.v. saline to correct volume depletion, potassium).
2. Moderate poisoning (< 500 mg/l AND acidosis OR < 750 mg/l alone) – alkaline diuresis (monitor CVP and give sodium bicarbonate to produce urine pH of 8–8.5).
3. Severe poisoning (< 750 mg/l AND renal impairment OR < 900 mg/l) – charcoal haemoperfusion or haemodialysis (ICU).

Some general measures would include:

- Gastric aspiration/lavage
- Activated charcoal orally
- Tepid sponging (hyperpyrexia)
- Vit K for hypoprothrombinaemia.

SUGGESTIONS FOR FURTHER PRACTICE

Self-poisoning is a medical emergency frequently seen by house officers. You need to know the features, investigations and management of the commonly taken drugs:

- Paracetamol
- Opiates
- Tricyclic antidepressants
- Benzodiazepines.

DATA 7	**Weight gain and hypertension**
Level:	***
Setting:	Structured oral with examiner
Time:	10 min

TASK

E – *You are the house officer for medicine. You are asked to see a patient on the Programmed-Investigation Unit. She is a 27-year-old woman who gives a history of putting on weight and her General Practitioner has found that her blood pressure has been increasing. You measure it and find it to be 170/110 mmHg, which is similar to the nurses' readings. Her urea and electrolytes have come back.*

Urea	6.5 mmol/l
Creat	93 µmol/l
Na	134 mmol/l
K	3.1 mmol/l

E – *What diagnoses are you thinking about to explain the history, examination and investigation findings and why?*

RESPONSE

The key skill or urea and electrolyte interpretation is discussed in Data 1. In this patient, the hypokalaemia, increased weight and hypertension suggests a number of diagnoses:

- Cushing's disease (most likely)
- Diuretic therapy for hypertension (does not account for weight change)
- Conn's syndrome (no weight change)
- Oral contraceptive pill (does not account for hypokalaemia)
- Alcohol (does not account for hypokalaemia).

E – *You have been asked to do a dexamethasone suppression test. Why is dexamethasone used? The results are given below:*

	Time	
Day 1 Serum cortisol	00:00	1020 nmol/l
	9:00	990 nmol/l

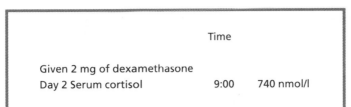

	Time	
Given 2 mg of dexamethasone		
Day 2 Serum cortisol	9:00	740 nmol/l

The dexamethasone is used to suppress ACTH and hence cortisol by negative feedback. It does not cross-react with laboratory assay of cortisol.

E – *What is your diagnosis? What would you look for on examination? What would you do next?*

The results show loss of diurnal variation of cortisol with persistent high readings despite dexamethasone. This again points to Cushing's disease. On examination, you might find:

- Moon face, plethoric complexion, subconjuctival oedema, acne and hirsutism in woman
- Thin skin, purpura
- Buffalo hump on trunk, centripetal obesity, purple striae ('lemon on stick')
- Limb muscle wasting and weakness.

It is impossible to distinguish clinically between Cushing's caused by pituitary adenoma or an adrenal tumour. Ectopic ACTH secretion from malignant tumours presents quite differently because the patients are very ill, wasted and heavily pigmented. Having demonstrated suppressible hypercortisolism, the next step is to measure plasma ACTH. If this is suppressed, the presumptive diagnosis is an adrenal adenoma, which can be confirmed by abdominal CT or MR scanning. If ACTH is unsuppressed, the patient may have either an ectopic (non-malignant) or pituitary source of ACTH. MR scanning of the pituitary may show an adenoma and MR or CT scan of the thorax may show an occult carcinoid tumour.

Most patients with 'high-ACTH Cushing's' will also need bilateral simultaneous inferior petrosal sinus sampling with corticotrophin-releasing hormone (CRH) stimulation.

SUGGESTIONS FOR FURTHER PRACTICE

Interpretation of either static or dynamic tests of endocrine/metabolic function requires detailed knowledge of hormonal control coupled with links to how dysfunction might present clinically. You should revise hyper- and hypo-function of:

- Anterior and posterior pituitary
- Thyroid
- Gonad
- Pancreas
- Parathyroid.

DATA 8	**Acute arthropathy**
Level:	***
Setting:	Structured oral
Time:	10 min

TASK

E – *You are looking after Freda Ward who has come into the ward because of severely painful hands. I would like you to look at the picture of her hands and tell me what you see and what you think the diagnosis is.*

RESPONSE

The core skill of hand examination is discussed in Examination 22. In this case, the patient has an asymmetrical arthropathy predominantly affecting the proximal inter-phalangeal joints, but probably also the distal interphalangeal joints. Given the pain, there is probably an acute inflammatory component.

The differential diagnosis includes rheumatoid arthritis (but this would be symmetrical) and acute osteoarthropathy (but usually predominantly distal joints). Psoriatic arthropathy is possible and you should tell the examiner that you would look for nail changes (pitting and nail bed separation – onycholyis) and skin patches. The other differential diagnosis is urate arthropathy.

E – *What would you do now?*

On this basis, you could investigate with:

● Plain radiographs of hands (erosions)

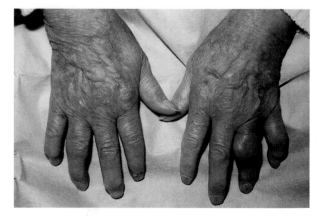

Figure 5.5

- Rheumatoid factor
- Urate levels
- Full blood count and ESR (normochromic normocytic anaemia).

E – *Routine blood tests were carried out, and this report came back from the Haematology Laboratory. How do you interpret it? How does it relate to the hand problem? What would be your management?*

Full blood count

Freda Ward d.o.b. 12/12/21

Hb	81 g/l
MCV	82 fl
WCC	83.4 × 10^9/l
Neutrophils	2.0
Lymphocytes	81.4
Platelets	43 × 10^9/l

The core skill of full blood count interpretation is discussed in data 5. Here, it shows a normochromic anaemia, thrombocytopenia and a very high white cell count. The most likely diagnosis is lymphatic leukaemia. You would need a film to distinguish between acute and chronic leukaemia; the presence of blast cells would indicate that it was acute.

The link between arthropathy and the leukaemia is the increased turnover of white cells leading to high urate and gouty arthropathy. You should also consider a septic arthropathy in association with immuno-suppression, but that usually involves just a single joint. The management of acute gout is with a non-steroidal anti-inflammatory drug to suppress the inflammation, then allopurinol to reduce uric acid formation. However, the most important action is to refer to a haematologist.

SUGGESTION FOR FURTHER PRACTICE

Make sure you can:

- Interpret large joint radiographs (hips and knees) and radiographs of the hands – particularly for erosions.
- Interpret basic immunology – ANF, RF, anti-neutrophil cytoplasmic antibody, anti-phospholipid antibodies, and antibodies to ENA, Jo and La.

CHAPTER 6

Procedure skills

Introduction

Procedures lend themselves well to testing in OSCE exams because they involve manual skills that can be tested objectively, often using an anatomical model or other form of simulation. Do not allow yourself to believe, however, that manual dexterity is all you need to do well in a procedure station. Clinical competence is a complex amalgam and the manual skill is rarely an end in its own right. Put differently, manual dexterity is necessary but not sufficient for clinical competence. Consider, for example, one of the most basic procedures, venepuncture (Procedure 13, page 227). To perform it without talking to the patient appropriately would be, at the least, a discourtesy and, at worst, a criminal assault. On top of that, it would be inexcusable not to know which tube the blood should go into for which test and why. You would look pretty foolish to put blood for measurement of the international normalised ratio (INR, a measurement of the adequacy of anticoagulation) into an orange-capped tube that contains heparin as an anticoagulant. And having taken the blood, you would look silly if you had no idea what an INR result of 9 means.[1]

PROCEDURE SKILLS

All procedures are like venepuncture in having the following components: the basic procedure, the associated communication skill, the contextual knowledge that underpins and surrounds the skill and the attitudes that allow you to use the skill appropriately.

Knowledge

- You need to understand the indications for performing the procedure, which may be quite complex (see Procedure 9: Blood transfusion).
- To be fluent and dextrous at performing the procedure, you need to memorise the sequence of steps.
- If there are choices to be made while performing it, you need good understanding to decide how to perform it in a particular situation (e.g. Procedure 16: Death certification).
- Basic knowledge of physiology and anatomy is often needed; take, for example, diagnostic pleural aspiration (Procedure 4). You cannot perform the procedure safely without knowing how the nerves and vessels lie in relation to the upper and lower rib margins (page 200).
- If it is a diagnostic procedure, you must know how to interpret the result. No examiner will take kindly to a candidate who is expert at inserting a lumbar puncture needle but cannot tell whether or not the patient has meningitis from the CSF analysis.
- If it is a therapeutic procedure, you need to know how to use the drug in

---

186   [1] Severe over-anticoagulation.

question. You may, for example, be called upon to give chemotherapy, calcium gluconate or antibiotics intravenously. The procedure is similar, but the contextual knowledge is very different.

Communication

Unless the patient is unconscious, you will need to use all the skills to build a relationship, understand his point of view, and recognise and respond to his emotions that are covered in Chapter 7. Good communication distinguishes a student who cares about patients from one who does not, and some marks will always be reserved for the quality of your communication skills. There is a legal and ethical dimension to communication. In all but dire emergencies, you may not perform a procedure without prior consent. The skill of obtaining consent, including how to give effective explanations, is covered in Chapter 7, Communication 5: Endoscopy (page 258) and Communication 7: Lumbar puncture (page 265).

The following points are common to all procedures:

- Obtain consent: That should not be obtained by a rhetorical question such as: *You don't mind if I take blood* …. It should be phrased: *May I take blood?* Do not proceed without a positive answer.
- Explain: You must explain what you are about to do (see Communication 6: Explain 24-h urine collection, page 262, for a description of the skill of explaining) but keep it short and clear and don't waste time. Students who lack confidence will give themselves away by lingering over wordy explanations rather than getting on with the job. In Procedure 4: Pleural aspiration, for example, you might say: *This test involves numbing the skin with local anaesthetic and then passing a needle through your skin and taking off a sample of fluid. You will feel a needle-prick as the anaesthetic needle penetrates the skin and then a little stinging as the anaesthetic is injected. It should certainly be no more painful than having a blood test, and you may feel very little more than pressure on your skin.*
- Maintain a dialogue with the patient as you go along: explain what you are doing and check their willingness for you to proceed.
- Be sensitive to how the patient feels: a competent but gentle manner coupled with sensitivity to discomfort and willingness to hear questions or concerns will be highly rated by patients and examiners.
- End appropriately: 'sign-off' pleasantly and courteously, and give the patient the chance to say or ask anything.

Often, you will be asked to perform a procedure on an anatomical model. Volunteer these important points about communication without waiting to be asked. You may be asked to talk to the examiner as if they were the patient (e.g. Procedure 13: Venepuncture). No matter how odd it feels, show the examiner your skills as a communicator.

Attitudes

In this context, attitudes straddle communication skills and contextual knowledge.

Take, for example, blood transfusion (Procedure 9). The UK General Medical Council states that one of the duties of a doctor is to 'treat every patient politely and considerately' and 'listen to patients and respect their views'. If the patient is a Jehovah's witness whose life is in danger (Attitude 3: A difficult haematemesis), your task will be to communicate in such a way that the problem can be discussed rationally. It will be hard to do so if you do not believe they have the right to refuse a blood transfusion. You need, also, to understand the ethical and legal principles that guide decision-making in this tricky situation.

Psychomotor skill

Manual skills are acquired by demonstration, followed by supervised and unsupervised practice until they become second nature. As has been explained above, knowledge plays a surprisingly large part in acquiring the skill. A person who is struggling to master a complex skill may find that it is not their manual dexterity that is at fault at all. A good explanation or study of a textbook may make the skill fall into place.

PERFORMING IN THE EXAMINATION SETTING

A common point of concern for students is whether to talk through procedures as they go along. Sometimes examiners will instruct you to do so (e.g. Procedure 7: Urethral catheterisation). Otherwise, your choice is to remain silent and make the structure of your procedure very obvious, or punctuate your performance with a statement of important points (particularly regarding the patient's comfort). The latter is probably the best approach but do not waffle about the obvious: *I am about to open the catheterisation pack* does not need to be stated and gives the impression of uncertainty. Emphasise key aspects of the procedure. A statement like: *I will inject about 5 ml of water and check that it is not painful to the patient before fully inflating the balloon* shows you are aware that the balloon may lodge in the urethra and are concerned about its consequences to the patient.

THE STATIONS

Six stations test diagnostic procedures. Each of them calls on you to interpret data. Nine stations test your therapeutic skills; six are therapeutic in their own right (e.g. urinary catheterisation) and three are procedures that allow you to give one of a number of different types of therapy (e.g. writing a prescription, intravenous injection). Finally, certification of death is an example of a complex clinical management skill. Not all skills can be covered in this book. You would be well advised to observe what other skills house officers are called upon to perform and be ready to encounter them in an examination.

HOW TO REVISE FOR PROCEDURE STATIONS

Syllabus

In Manchester, we identified 70 procedures, laboratory skills, therapeutic skills or complex clinical management skills that our graduates should be able to perform at the time of qualification. Some are everyday skills that house officers have to perform without supervision. Others are called upon infrequently, but in an emergency when there is nobody to supervise. Some are basic and lend themselves to testing in an OSCE. Others are more complex. If your medical school has not defined the procedural skills that it expects of you, it would be sensible to read this chapter and then see if you can devise a list of what is likely to be covered in your examinations. Even if you are wrong, it will pay dividends in building your clinical competence!

Preparation

Ask yourself these questions:

Knowledge
What are the indications for performing the skill?
Do I know the steps of the procedure?
Does the procedure need to be 'tailored' to the individual patient in any way?
Is there any underpinning anatomy or physiology that I should revise?
Is there an associated task of data interpretation?
Is there associated therapeutic knowledge?

Communication
Do I understand the general principles of communication associated with procedural skills?
Could I explain the procedure clearly enough to a patient to obtain informed consent?
How can I be sure to use good communication skills when performing it?

Attitudes
Are there any important ethical or legal issues associated with this procedure?
Am I clear about my own attitudes towards and knowledge of those issues?

Skill
Can I perform the skill dextrously and with confidence?

Practice

There is a hierarchy of ways of developing the skill:

- On an anatomical model
- On a fellow student (for a few procedure skills)
- On a patient, supervised
- On a patient, unsupervised.

The student who will perform best in an OSCE is the one who has pushed their performance as far up this hierarchy as possible. There is no substitute for self-directed practice!

PROCEDURE 1	**Record an ECG**
Level:	*
Setting:	Healthy young man lying on a couch stripped to the waist and with bare ankles; extension into ECG interpretation
Time:	5 min

TASK

E – *Please use this 12-lead ECG machine to record an ECG on this patient.*

RESPONSE

This is not pass/fail knowledge but it will impress the examiner if you know that 1 mV causes a vertical deflection of 10 mm (2 large squares) and that the normal paper speed is 25 mm/s (5 large squares per second). These figures become important if the calibration is changed; for example, the sensitivity may be halved in a patient with very high voltage complexes caused by left ventricular hypertrophy, or the paper speed may be slowed to interpret a complex tachy-dysrhythmia.

Core skill: Recording an ECG

1. Introduce yourself, explain what you would like to do and obtain consent (Introduction to Procedures; page 187).

2. Attach the limb leads to the four limbs; place pads or electrode jelly under each electrode as you position it.

3. Ensure good skin contact without discomfort.

4. Position the chest leads as follows:
   V1 Fourth intercostal space at right sternal border
   V2 Fourth intercostal space at left sternal border
   V3 Midway between V2 and V4
   V4 Fifth intercostal space in the midclavicular line
   V5 Anterior axillary line at same horizontal level as V4
   V6 Mid-axillary line at same horizontal level as V4 and V5.

5. Switch on the machine and record the ECG.

E – *Please report this ECG.*

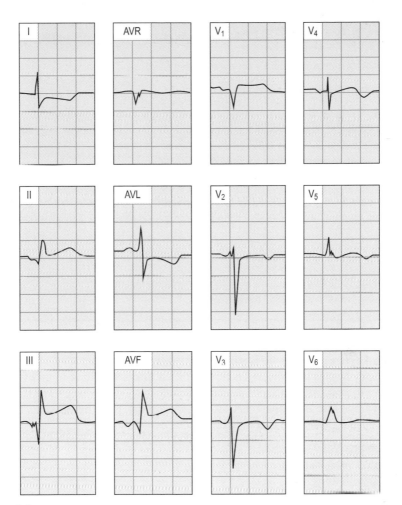

Figure 6.1

If you are hazy about the common patterns of disease on the ECG, you should revise them. This ECG shows ST segment elevation > 1 mm in leads III and aVF with similar, though less marked, changes in II. There is T wave inversion in leads V_2 to V_5. This is the characteristic picture of an acute inferior infarct; you can tell that it is acute because the ST segments are elevated and T wave inversion has not yet developed in the inferior leads (II, III and aVF). The T wave changes across the chest leads are 'reciprocal'. An astute observer will note that the P waves are inverted in the inferior leads and V_2 to V_4, with a short PR interval, indicating a nodal rhythm.

SUGGESTIONS FOR FURTHER PRACTICE

Go to an OSCE exam prepared to interpret ECGs as well as record them. The best way of learning ECG interpretation is to shadow an acute medical team for 24 hours of emergency 'take', record several ECGs, and have a stab at interpreting

Core skill: Reading an ECG

Read ECGs systematically, in the following order:

1. Scan the ECG quickly to see if any gross abnormalities catch your attention.

2. Rate: If regular, divide 300 by the number of large squares between two successive QRS complexes; if irregular, divide 900 by the number of large squares between four successive QRS complexes. A normal heart rate is 60–100/min, or 5–3 large squares between two successive complexes.

3. Rhythm and conduction: Check for regularity of the complexes, the relation between P waves and successive QRS complexes (The PR interval; normal < 5 small squares), and the width of the QRS complexes (normal < 3 small squares).

4. Axis: If the S wave is greater than the R wave in lead I, there is right axis deviation. If the S wave is greater than the R wave in lead II, there is left axis deviation.

5. Configuration of the QRST complexes.

the ECG of every patient who is admitted. You might ask a senior Coronary Care Nurse if they have a teaching collection of ECGs and are willing to go over some of them with you. Alternatively, attach yourself to the Coronary Care Unit for a couple of days and examine every ECG you can lay your hands on. These are some abnormal ECGs that you may be shown in an exam:

- Acute myocardial infarction
- Left ventricular hypertrophy
- Atrial fibrillation
- Supraventricular tachycardia
- Ventricular tachycardia
- Ventricular fibrillation
- Heart block.

PROCEDURE 2	**Intravenous injection**
Level:	**
Setting:	Structured viva and skills test using an anatomical arm, extended into clinical management
Time:	10 min

TASK

E – *It is 03:00 A.M. You are a house officer. A 75-year-old man is brought into the resuscitation room of Casualty sitting bolt upright and gasping for breath. His wife tells you that he has not seen a doctor for 20 years and is on no regular treatment. Unusually, he complained of indigestion after tea yesterday. He became breathless during sleep with an audible wheeze. He developed a cough and brought up white frothy sputum tinged with blood. You listen quickly to his chest and hear inspiratory crackles and a wheeze. What are you going to do?*

RESPONSE

With an acute onset of nocturnal dyspnoea and wheeze, the main differential is between left ventricular failure (LVF) and airways obstruction. He has no previous history of airways obstruction. The 'indigestion' may well have been cardiac pain. Everything points towards LVF, causing 'cardiac asthma' (bronchospasm secondary to LVF). Whatever the diagnosis, you should:

- Give 100% oxygen; he has no history of COPD so there is no danger that a high concentration of inspired oxygen will suppress respiration.
- Put in a venous cannula.
- Do an immediate ECG to exclude myocardial infarction, or a dysrhythmia.
- Arrange for a chest X-ray once he has received emergency treatment and is a little better.

E – *What drug treatment should you give?*

With a working diagnosis of LVF, your choice is between one or more of the following drugs, given intravenously:

- A loop diuretic • A nitrate • An opiate.

The patient is extremely distressed so it would be wise to give diamorphine with an anti-emetic (e.g. prochlorperazine) by the intravenous route. You will need to give a second drug; a nitrate will relieve LVF as effectively or more so than a loop diuretic but the use of loop diuretics in this situation is time-honoured so it is probably safest to say that you will give intravenous frusemide or bumetanide.

E – *What dose of frusemide will you give?*

It will show that you are clinically experienced if you can quote a drug dose but it is dangerous to do so unless you are absolutely sure that you are right. A good compromise would be to say that 40 mg is the appropriate dose but, at this stage of your career, you would always double-check against the British National Formulary.

E – *Here is a vial of frusemide; let us assume that you have had difficulty siting a venous cannula. Please show me how you would give frusemide 40 mg by direct intravenous injection.*

Core skill: Intravenous drug injection

According to the drug in question, you have to select between:

- Direct intravenous administration; if a very rapid response is required (e.g. diuretic for LVF).

- Infusion in a drip bag; for drugs that have to be given slowly (e.g. antibiotics or cytotoxics).

- Administration by a syringe pump; where a steady plasma concentration is needed (e.g. insulin or heparin).

- Administration through a central – as opposed to peripheral – venous cannula; for drugs that are irritant to veins (e.g. amiodarone or dopamine).

The procedure for a direct intravenous injection is:

1. Introduce yourself, explain what you would like to do and obtain consent (Introduction to Procedures; page 187).

2. Check the vial carefully for the name of the drug and concentration.

3. Attach a green (21 G) needle to a 5 ml syringe.

4. Assuming the concentration is 10 mg/ml, draw a little more than 4 ml into the syringe.

5. Hold the syringe and needle vertically, with the needle pointing upwards. Tap the syringe so that air bubbles rise to the top.

6. Gently advance the plunger so that the syringe contains exactly 4 ml and the air has been expelled.

7. Discard the needle and attach a fresh green (21 G) needle.

8. Position and tighten the tourniquet and do a venepuncture (Procedure 12: Basic life support).

9. Draw a little blood back into the syringe.

10. Once you are satisfied that the needle is well positioned in the vein, loosen the tourniquet and gently advance the plunger.

E – *How quickly can the dose be given?*

The British National Formulary specifies that the rate of injection should not exceed 4 mg/min, although few house officers give it as slowly as that. The examiner is probing to find out if you know that frusemide is a drug which can be given relatively quickly.

E – *Please give me one example of an emergency drug which has to be given by <u>slow</u> intravenous injection.*

The classic is calcium gluconate for the acute management of hypocalcaemia – <u>10 ml</u> of <u>10%</u> solution over <u>10 minutes</u>. There are many others, particularly anti-dysrhythmics, which are given in emergencies, but can cause asystole or ventricular fibrillation if given as a rapid bolus.

E – *How quickly would you give an intravenous bolus of potassium chloride containing 20 mmol of potassium?*

This is a trick question (something you should not really be faced with). Potassium must NEVER be given as a bolus injection. It is given in a 500 or 1000 ml bag of intravenous fluid. Very exceptionally, a more concentrated solution may be given through a syringe pump or in a small drip bag but there is such a great risk of causing cardiac arrest if the infusion inadvertently runs too fast that this cannot be recommended in any but exceptional circumstances.

E – *You have given diamorphine 5 mg, prochlorperazine 12.5 mg and frusemide 40 mg. Thirty minutes later, the patient is still very breathless and ill. What should you do now?*

You should reassess the patient, measure his blood gases and call for senior help. Your therapeutic options are to do one or more of the following:

- Repeat the frusemide and increase the dose (e.g. to 80 mg).
- Start a nitrate infusion as well.
- Request an intensive care admission with a view to:
  - Giving more diamorphine (which could cause respiratory failure).
  - Treating any underlying cardiac problem (e.g. a dysrhythmia).
  - Inotrope therapy (e.g. if he is hyopotensive).
  - Ventilation.

SUGGESTIONS FOR FURTHER PRACTICE

This station will 'find out' the student who has never done a night on call. If you work with a duty house officer, you will have the chance to observe the

PROCEDURE SKILLS

195

emergency management of this common situation and may be allowed to administer treatment. Helpful though it is to learn skills on anatomical models in the safety of a skills lab, examiners will be canny at spotting people who have not gained REAL experience and OSCE examinations are set up to test applied, as opposed to theoretical, knowledge.

PROCEDURE 3	**Advanced life support**
Level:	★★★
Setting:	A training defibrillator and resuscitation mannequin
Time:	5 min

TASK

E – *Please imagine that this person has been brought into the Casualty resuscitation room having collapsed. Basic life support was given. He is now being ventilated and given cardiac massage and has a venous cannula in place. This is his rhythm strip. Please demonstrate how you would respond.*

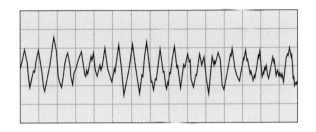

Figure 6.2

RESPONSE

This strip shows ventricular fibrillation (VF). It is not sufficient just to recognise the rhythm, although you will fail the exam if you cannot recognise it and describe how to treat it. You must communicate a sense of urgency in your response and not wait to be prompted because a delay of minutes will affect the patient's chance of survival. This is what you should demonstrate to the examiner:

- Charge the defibrillator to 200 J.
- Position one electrode pad below the right clavicle in the mid-clavicular line and the other just outside the cardiac apex (between left mid and anterior axillary lines).
- Apply paddles.
- Alert other personnel that you are going to defibrillate.
- Defibrillate.
- Check monitor. If still in VF, defibrillate again at 200 J.
- Check monitor. If still in VF, defibrillate again at 360 J.
- Check monitor. Give cardiopulmonary resuscitation (CPR) for 1 minute.
- If still in VF:
  - Give adrenaline 1 mg intravenously.
  - Check adequacy of ventilation and oxygenation.
- Repeat 3 cycles of: checking that the patient remains in VF; defibrillation at

197

360 J; CPR for 1 min; and further adrenaline 1 mg. This complete cycle should be done in no more than 3 min.

E – *When will you stop defibrillating?*

- If the waveform changes to:
  - Sinus tachycardia or some other rhythm which is likely to support a cardiac output.
  - Asystole.

E – *How can you assure safety during the use of a defibrillator?*

- Remove dermal nitrate patches (which may explode!).
- Ensure the paddles are a minimum of 15 cm away from any pacemaker box.
- Do not apply electrode jelly carelessly or spill fluids close to the defibrillation site.
- Keep wet clothing away from the paddles.
- Ensure that no-one touches the patient or bed during defibrillation.
- Shout 'stand clear' before defibrillating.

E – *You have completed three cycles of defibrillation, and still the patient is in VF; what now?*

Consider and treat any possible reversible causes:

- Inadequate oxygenation.
- Hyperkalaemia: measure serum potassium; give calcium gluconate if severe hyperkalaemia is suspected or proven.
- Metabolic acidosis: check blood gases and give bicarbonate if the patient is acidotic.
- Hypovolaemia: give intravenous colloid if there is evidence of severe volume depletion.
- Poisoning, tension pneumothorax, cardiac tamponade, thromboembolism.

Give an intravenous anti-arrhythmic such as lignocaine, bretylium or amiodarone.

E – *Suppose the patient were in asystole when the monitor was first applied, what would you do to treat the arrhythmia?*

- Give atropine 3 mg and adrenaline 1 mg.

E – *What factors predict whether a patient with cardiac arrest will survive?*

- Effective provision of basic life support (see Procedure 12).
- Immediate defibrillation of VF or VT.
- The outcome is much better with VF/VT than other dysrhythmias.

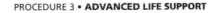

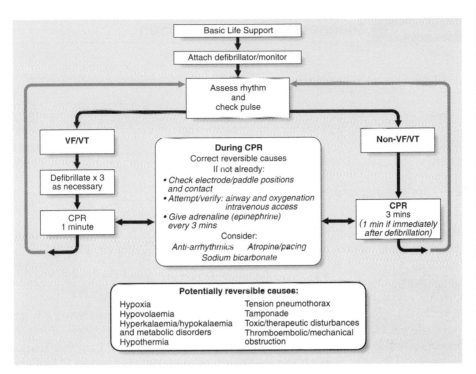

Figure 6.3 Advanced life support. This figure has been adapted with kind permission of the publishers from Br Med J (1998) 316: 1863–1869

SUGGESTIONS FOR FURTHER PRACTICE

Many hospitals have a training defibrillator which allows you to familiarise yourself with the technique in safety. You must, before qualification, attend cardiac arrests as a member of the team, and practise basic and advanced life support in real situations (see Procedure 12). You must be absolutely confident at both procedures on resuscitation models and be able to state the above management guidelines clearly and confidently.

PROCEDURE 4 — Diagnostic pleural aspiration

Level:	**
Setting:	X-ray viewing box and middle-aged male volunteer stripped to the waist, extended into data interpretation
Time:	10 min

TASK

E – *What does this radiograph show?*

The examiner shows you the radiograph in Examination 5: Heart examination, p. 94. See Data 2 for the core skill of interpreting a chest radiograph.

RESPONSE

You should have no difficulty recognising that the radiograph shows a large right pleural effusion. Since the examiner asked you what it shows, the best response would be to state the diagnosis. A direct answer will gain you marks for competence. Go through the routine of giving a detailed report if you are unsure, but you will not give a good impression and it will cost you time.

E – *Please demonstrate on this volunteer how you would perform a diagnostic pleural aspiration; when it comes to the point of injecting him, please just describe the procedure.*

(See Core skill: Diagnostic pleural aspiration)

E – *Suppose you did all that, introduced the needle to its full length and no fluid came back. Why might that be?*

- You chose too high an interspace.
- The pleura are thickened by fibrosis or tumour infiltration.
- The pleural fluid is viscid; it may be fibrinous or purulent (empyema).

E – *What would you do?*

- Repeat the procedure one interspace down.
- Use a larger needle if you suspected there was viscid fluid.

E – *You're still having no success; what next?*

- Ask a radiologist to do an ultrasound scan, check that there is fluid, see if it is loculated, and either direct you to a better position for your pleural aspiration or do it themself.

Core skill: Diagnostic pleural aspiration

1. Introduce yourself, explain what you would like to do and obtain consent (Introduction to Procedures; page 187).

2. Assemble equipment: sterile pack, gloves, antiseptic solution, 2 or 5 ml syringe for local anaesthetic, 20 ml syringe to aspirate fluid, orange (25 G) and green (21 G) needles, vial of local anaesthetic, plain sterile tubes and tubes for specific tests (e.g. cytology, glucose).

3. Ask the patient to sit upright and lean forwards with their arms crossed in front of them. The patient should have something firm to lean against; e.g. sit up on the bed with a bed table in front of them, or sit back-to-front astride a chair and lean on pillows on the back of the chair or a high table. This position elevates the scapulae and gives you good access to the lower thorax posteriorly.

4. Ensure that the patient is relatively comfortable and maintain a dialogue with them throughout the procedure.

5. Percuss the right lower thorax posteriorly and identify the area of dullness caused by the effusion; delineate the upper limit of dullness.

6. Palpate the margins of the two ribs that form the interspace below the top of the effusion.

7. Wash your hands and wear gloves. Use sterile technique.

8. Clean the skin with antiseptic solution, using cotton wool held with forceps.

9. Draw up local anaesthetic and infiltrate the skin with the orange (25 G) needle.

10. Introduce the needle about 10 cm lateral to the midline just above the lower of the two ribs (remember that the neurovascular bundle, which you must avoid, runs along the lower border of the upper rib).

11. Infiltrate down to pleura with the green (21 G) needle, always aspirating before injecting anaesthetic solution. You may feel the parietal pleura 'give' as you advance the needle, at which point pleural fluid may flush back into the syringe.

12. Attach a green needle to the 20 ml syringe and introduce it perpendicular to the skin, just above the rib which forms the lower margin of the interspace, following the track of the local anaesthetic. Penetrate the parietal pleura and aspirate 20 ml fluid

13. Withdraw the needle and cover the entry site with a dry gauze dressing.

14. Send the aspirated fluid in appropriately labelled sterile containers to the laboratory.

E – *You aspirate successfully. The pleural fluid is pale in appearance and has a protein concentration of 20 g/l. The plasma total protein concentration is 70 g/l. How do you interpret that result?*

Even if you were caught unawares by this question, you could improve your performance by taking a few seconds to think through and structure your answer. Basic clinical knowledge will give you the six headings in the Core skill box, below and much of the rest of the table follows logically.

Core skill: Interpretation of pleural fluid

Colour
- Pale, serous fluid suggests transudate or inflammatory exudate
- Blood-staining suggests infarct or tumour
- Turbidity suggests infection
- Chylous fluid suggests malignant lymphatic obstruction.

Biochemistry
- Total protein > 30 g/l or pleural fluid total protein > 50% of blood total protein indicates inflammatory exudate
- Glucose low in rheumatoid or effusions related to pneumonia
- Amylase raised in effusions associated with pancreatitis.

Microscopy
- Gram stain may identify bacterial infection
- ZN stain specific but not sensitive for tuberculosis.

Culture
- Fluid must be cultured for aerobic and anaerobic infections, and tuberculosis.

Cytology
- May identify malignant pleural disease, although pleural biopsy is much more informative.

Immunology
- Rheumatoid factor may be positive in rheumatoid effusions.

The pleural fluid in this case is clearly a transudate; in other words, an ultrafiltrate of plasma resulting from increased venous pressure (heart failure) or reduced colloid osmotic pressure (hypoalbuminaemia). The causes of hypoalbuminaemia are reduced albumin synthesis (e.g. liver failure or severe systemic illness) or increased albumin loss (e.g. nephrotic syndrome).

A way to score high marks in this station would be to refer back to the original radiograph without being prompted and comment on the presence or absence of signs of heart failure, e.g.:

- Cardiomegaly

- Alveolar oedema
- Upper lobe venous diversion.

SUGGESTIONS FOR FURTHER PRACTICE

Diagnostic pleural aspiration is a procedure that you might have a chance to perform before qualification and must certainly have observed. A chest ward is the best place to gain experience. As with other diagnostic procedures, don't allow yourself to be so mesmerised by the procedure that you forget to learn how to interpret the result. You will be expected to be able to interpret data in a skills station, and may also be questioned on pleural fluid analysis in an MCQ. Follow through patients whose pleural aspirations you observe and see how the results are used in their management.

PROCEDURE 5	**Write a prescription**
Level:	***
Setting:	'Viva' format extended into clinical management
Time:	5 min

TASK

E – *A 29-year-old woman who has previously had excellent health is admitted under your care with a 7-day history of malaise, feverishness and cough. She has pleuritic pain in her left axilla. Her temperature is 38.5°C. You find an area of dullness in the left axilla with bronchial breath sounds. She is uncomfortable but able to joke with you as you examine her. She has no known allergies. What do you think is the diagnosis?*

RESPONSE

This is obviously pneumonia and you should say that without beating around the bush. You would gain extra credit for saying *community-acquired* pneumonia (because *hospital-acquired pneumonia* has a different spectrum of pathogens and is treated differently). Ordinarily, you would offer a differential diagnosis but there scarcely is one here. Since the examiner is testing your knowledge, you might volunteer the likely causative organisms.

E – *What do you think the infecting organism might be?*

- *Streptococcus pneumoniae* (50–80%)
- An atypical organism (up to 20%).
  - *Mycoplasma pneumoniae.*
  - *Legionella* spp.
- *Haemophilus* spp.
- A virus:
  - *Influenza.*
  - *Staphylococcus aureus.*

E – *What antibiotic therapy would you give?*

There are really two questions here:

- Oral or intravenous therapy?
- Which drug(s)?

Intravenous therapy with ceftriaxone, for example, is much more expensive than oral therapy and unnecessary for many patients. It is best reserved for those with poor prognostic features. A patient with two or more of these features has severe pneumonia:

- Respiratory rate > 30/min.
- Plasma urea > 7 mmol/l.
- Diastolic blood pressure < 60 mmHg.

The final sentence of the examiner's original instruction gives a strong hint that this patient is well enough to be treated orally. It will come across well if you reason your way towards oral therapy.

E – *What oral antibiotic or antibiotics would you choose?*

A good first-line choice of antibiotic would be amoxycillin. Atypical pneumonia does not respond to penicillins and is so common that many clinicians would give a macrolide (erythromycin) as well. This should certainly be added if the patient does not respond well to amoxycillin.

E – *What information about a patient (and now I am talking in general terms, not just about this woman with pneumonia) would you write on the cover page of a hospital prescription chart?* (Hands you a blank prescription chart.) *Please write a hospital prescription for amoxycillin 500 mg three times daily by mouth to start today.*

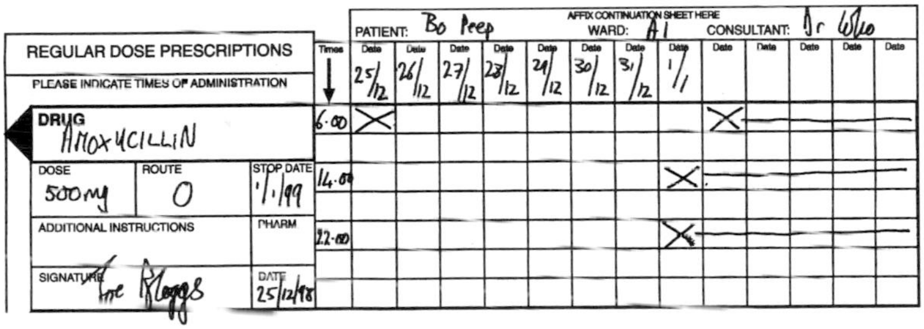
REGULAR DOSE PRESCRIPTIONS
PLEASE INDICATE TIMES OF ADMINISTRATION
PATIENT: Bo Peep
AFFIX CONTINUATION SHEET HERE
WARD: A1
CONSULTANT: Dr Who
DRUG: AMOXYCILLIN
DOSE: 500mg
ROUTE: O
STOP DATE: 1/1/99
ADDITIONAL INSTRUCTIONS
PHARM
SIGNATURE: Joe Bloggs
DATE: 25/12/98
Times: 6.00, 14.00, 22.00
Date: 25/12, 26/12, 27/12, 28/12, 29/12, 30/12, 31/12, 1/1

Figure 6.4

SUGGESTIONS FOR FURTHER PRACTICE

Pharmacists are experts on drug therapy and prescribing who spend much of their lives rectifying the mistakes of doctors. Ask your ward pharmacist to give you a tutorial on good prescribing habits, and on some more complex issues such as prescribing controlled drugs.

Core skill: Completing a prescription chart

Information to be written on the cover page of the chart:

1. Full and accurate identification details, including:
   Name
   Age
   Hospital number
   Ward
   Consultant.

2. Any allergies.

3. Details of any other treatments which the patient is receiving and for which there may be a separate chart, e.g.:
   Anticoagulants
   Insulin
   Diet.

A completed prescription is shown in Figure 6.4. The key features are:

4. Clear and legible handwriting, in ink.

5. Drug name in capitals.

6. Correct generic name of the drug.

7. Doses appropriately spaced through the day.

8. Dated.

9. Stop date specified (for an antibiotic); in this case, a 7-day course.

10. Legible signature.

PROCEDURE 6 — Nasogastric intubation

Level:	**
Setting:	Summative workplace assessment in which a student is asked to demonstrate the skill on a hospitalised female patient. A 16 F Ryle's tube (wide-bore nasogastric tube) and other equipment are provided
Time:	Unlimited

TASK

Pass a nasogastric tube.

RESPONSE

Communication aspects of the skill are covered in the introductory section of this chapter, page 187. This is an uncomfortable procedure so you need to acknowledge the discomfort and encourage the patient as well as show confidence in the skill.

Core skill: Pass a nasogastric tube

1. Introduce yourself, explain what you would like to do and obtain consent (Introduction to Procedures; page 187).

2. Ask the patient to sit on a chair or the edge of the bed with neck slightly flexed.

3. Wash your hands and put on gloves.

4. Measure the distance from the tip of the patient's nose to the ear lobe and from the ear lobe to the xiphisternum and mark that distance on the tube with tape.

5. Place the nasogastric tube, gauze, tube of KY jelly, Xylocaine spray and a glass of water with a straw on a clean surface adjacent to the patient.

6. Spray the nostril with Xylocaine.

7. Squirt jelly onto the gauze and lubricate the end section of the tube.

8. Pass the tube into the patient's nostril and along the floor of the nose into the nasopharynx.

9. When the patient is aware of the tube in the back of the throat, ask them to tilt their head forward and take sips of water through a straw.

10. Each time the patient swallows, advance the tube a few centimetres (so that the epiglottis is closed whenever the tube is advanced).

> **Core skill:** *(cont'd)*
>
> 11. If the patient coughs violently, pull the tube back a few centimetres.
>
> 12. Talk to the patient encouragingly throughout the procedure.
>
> 13. Once the tube is in the oesophagus, it should be possible to advance it quite rapidly into the stomach.
>
> 14. Check that the tube is in the correct position by injecting a small volume of air into it from a syringe and listening with a stethoscope.
>
> 15. Tape the tube to the patient's nose.

E – *What are the indications for putting in a Ryle's tube?*

The only reason for putting in a wide-bore nasogastric tube is to apply suction and aspirate stomach contents. Some indications are:

- To empty the stomach:
  - Before and after GI surgery
  - In intestinal obstruction
  - After trauma or in serious illness when there is a risk of aspiration.
- To aspirate stomach contents for diagnostic purposes:
  - To assess the progress of upper GI bleeding
  - After some forms of self-poisoning.

If a nasogastric tube is needed to feed the patient or give medications enterally, it should be a fine-bore tube which is:

- Softer and much less uncomfortable
- Less likely to cause oesophageal inflammation and stricture
- Able to stay in for a longer time (> 1 week).

E – *How does the insertion of a fine-bore tube differ from the procedure you have just done?*

Fine-bore tubes (e.g. 8 F gauge) have a guide wire to make them rigid enough to insert. Because the tube collapses when suction is applied to it, and is too fine to allow air to be bubbled briskly through it, it is only possible to prove that it is correctly positioned by X-raying the patient (the tube has a radio-opaque marker). This must ALWAYS be done before putting anything down the tube.

SUGGESTIONS FOR FURTHER PRACTICE

Although nurses usually put in Ryle's tubes, it should be part of your general training to learn the skill. As a house officer, you may be asked to take responsibility for positioning a fine-bore feeding tube so you would do well to learn the skill before qualification.

Urethral catheterisation

Level:	*
Setting:	Male anatomical model and trolley with catheterisation sterile pack
Time:	5 min

TASK

E – *Please pass a urethral catheter; describe how you would perform the procedure on a real patient as you go along.*

RESPONSE

The examiner has specifically asked you to talk through the procedure so pay particular attention to the suggestions on page 188.

Core skill: Urethral catheterisation

1. Introduce yourself, explain what you would like to do and obtain consent (Introduction to Procedures; page 187).

2. Lie the patient comfortably on his back with his legs slightly separated.

3. Choose a 16 F catheter.

4. Open the catheterisation pack, pour antiseptic into the receiver and put on gloves.

5. Clean the penis thoroughly, retract the prepuce and clean around the meatus.

6. Drape, so that only the penis is in the sterile field.

7. Hold the penis with a gauze swab.

8. Squeeze anaesthetic/lubricant jelly into the urethra and occlude it with pressure from the gauze.

9. Explain that you would allow at least 5 minutes for the anaesthetic to work.

10. Advance the catheter tip from its sleeve and introduce it into the urethra.

11. Advance the catheter using a 'no touch technique', or with sterile forceps, until the end-arm of the catheter is up to the meatus.

12. Inflate the balloon: inject about 5 ml of water and check that it does not cause pain before fully inflating it.

13. Attach the bag.

Core skill: *(cont'd)*

14. Gently extend the catheter into position.

15. Reposition the prepuce.

16. Record the volume of urine in the bag (residual volume).

E – *What are the indications for catheterisation?*

- Urinary retention.
- Incontinence.
- When a patient is temporarily incapacitated, e.g. after surgery or in severe illness:
  - GU surgery
  - Other major surgery
  - Severe illness, trauma, intensive care.
- To monitor urine output; e.g. in the management of acute renal failure.
- To give intra-vesical chemotherapy.
- Investigation, e.g. micturating cystourethrography.

E – *What are the contraindications?*

- Suspected urethral injury; the signs of this are perineal bruising and/or blood at the meatus.
- A history of urethral stricture or false passages.

Examiners are keen to see that students, as house officers, will know when they are out of their depth and be prepared to call for help. A good way of answering the question about contraindications would be: *If the patient had … I would discuss the problem with a senior colleague or urologist.*

E – *What are the complications of catheterisation?*

- Pain
- Infection
- Irritation and possibly stricture if a rubber (as opposed to silicone) catheter is left in place for more than 3 weeks.

E – *Suppose no urine came out?*

- Most likely the catheter is blocked with jelly. Flush it with saline.
- The catheter tip may be misplaced.
- There may be no urine in the bladder; for example, the patient is in acute renal failure and suprapubic tenderness was misattributed to bladder distension.

SUGGESTIONS FOR FURTHER PRACTICE

Master the technique of urethral catheterisation on an anatomical model as early as you can and become competent at doing it on real patients. Catheterisation is a humdrum task which house officers will be pleased to delegate to you but they will know that they cannot do so until they have supervised and checked that you are competent so there is a real incentive for them to help you develop this skill. If you clerk patients who have been admitted for surgery, they may gladly give consent for you to perform the procedure under general anaesthetic.

PROCEDURE SKILLS

PROCEDURE 8 | # Venous cannulation

Level:	**
Setting:	An anatomical arm. Sharps bin and venous cannulation tray provided. Giving set already run through. Extension into clinical management
Time:	5 min

TASK

E – *Imagine that this arm belongs to a woman with advanced chronic renal failure who has pneumonia, has been vomiting and is volume-depleted. Please put up a drip.*

Core skill: Venous cannulation

1. Introduce yourself, explain what you would like to do and obtain consent (Introduction to Procedures; page 187).

2. Select equipment from the tray:
   - 18 gauge venous cannula
   - Strips of tape to fix the cannula in place
   - Tourniquet
   - Gloves.

3. Check that the giving set is correctly run through; check what fluid is in the bag.

4. Position the arm and identify a suitable vein.

5. Check that the patient is willing for you to proceed.

6. Apply the tourniquet and re-check the vein.

7. Put on gloves.

8. Remove the cannula from its pack, using a 'no-touch technique'.

9. Explain to the patient what they will feel.

10. Stretch the skin, then insert the needle, bevel upwards.

11. When blood flushes back into the hub, advance the cannula off its needle.

12. Release the tourniquet.

13. Remove the needle and discard it in the sharps bin.

14. Press over the vein around the tip of the cannula and remove the cap.

15. Attach the giving set.

16. Fix the cannula and tubing securely in place with tape.

17. Adjust the drip to run slowly.

RESPONSE

See Procedure 13: Venepuncture, for some general points about venous access and hospital policies.

E – *Where is the best place to site a venous cannula?*

Although venous cannulation is a 'generic' skill that you learn early in your clinical training, remember that this station has been identified as a 'genitourinary' one, and at intermediate (**) level. Examiners will be looking for more than basic competence by this stage of your training. Usually, any large forearm vein is suitable for a venous cannula. It is best to stay away from the elbow and wrist if possible to minimise inconvenience and discomfort, and prevent the cannula being dislodged. However, the 'stem' of this station gave you the extra information that the patient has chronic renal failure. She may be a candidate for dialysis. Drips can thrombose veins, particularly if irritant solutions are infused. Her forearm veins may be needed for an arterio-venous shunt or fistula for haemodialysis so a thrombosed vein would be a disaster. A fistula or shunt is likely to be sited in the non-dominant arm for convenience. Avoid that arm completely, and avoid forearm veins in either arm if at all possible. You would gain marks by relating the later question to the information given to you in the original 'stem' without being prompted by the examiner.

E – *What fluid would you give?*

Fluid therapy is one of the basic responsibilities of house officers, and one that they often find difficult. However, some simple principles apply, as summarised in the core skill box.

SUGGESTIONS FOR FURTHER PRACTICE

Become thoroughly competent at venous cannulation during your clerkships. Remember that no patient goes through surgery without a drip so use surgical and anaesthetic attachments to practise the skill in theatre. Venous cannulae are of no use unless something is put through them. Learn about intravenous therapy by questioning the management of every patient that you see. The best place to learn fluid therapy is a renal ward.

PROCEDURE SKILLS

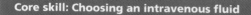

PROCEDURE SKILLS

Core skill: Choosing an intravenous fluid

1. Before prescribing, assess the patient's blood volume and general clinical condition (lying and standing pulse and blood pressure, hydration of the tongue and axilla, and jugular venous pressure lying at 45° and flat).

2. Check the renal function and electrolytes.

3. If the patient has lost blood, transfuse.

4. If in hypovolaemic shock, give colloid.

5. If in metabolic acidosis, consider giving bicarbonate but discuss with a senior colleague first.

6. If the serum sodium is very high or very low, consider giving hypotonic or hypertonic saline, but do not do so without senior supervision.

7. Otherwise, give an isotonic solution (5% dextrose, 0.9% saline or dextrose saline).

8. If the patient is volume-depleted, give saline. If euvolaemic, alternate dextrose and saline, or give dextrose saline.

9. Tailor the rate of fluid administration to the patient's measured or expected urinary loss, allowing an extra volume of about 0.5 l per 24 h for 'insensible' loss, and adjust this rate upwards or downwards to correct any pre-existing overload or deficit.

10. Give added potassium (e.g. 20 mmol/l), adjusted upwards or downwards to correct any abnormality of plasma potassium.

11. Watch the patient's jugular venous pressure, blood pressure, arterial pulse, urine flow, and urea and electrolytes to monitor the effect of your therapy.

PROCEDURE 9   **Blood transfusion**

Level:	***
Setting:	A structured viva extended into data interpretation (see linked Attitude 3: A difficult haematemesis)
Time:	10 min

TASK

The examiner hands you a card that reads as follows:

> Mrs Elsie Thomas, aged 74, was admitted under your
> care yesterday after a fall. She has osteoarthritis and
> takes occasional ibuprofen. She has noticed vague upper
> abdominal pain and lacked energy for the last three
> months. On examination, you noted some ankle swelling
> and the signs of her arthritis but found no other
> abnormal signs. Her blood count is as follows:
>
> Hb 80 g/l
> MVC 72 fl
> Platelets 240 × 10^9/l
> White cell count 8.0 × 10^9/l

E – *How do you interpret this information?*

RESPONSE

It may have struck you immediately that the patient is taking a non-steroidal anti-inflammatory drug and has a microcytic anaemia, making it very likely that she is bleeding from a peptic ulcer; however, you need to tackle the case systematically. A logical approach would be as follows:

1. The blood picture is grossly abnormal:
   She is very anaemic with a low mean cell volume. The platelets and white cell count are normal. The most likely diagnosis is iron deficiency anaemia.

Note that you were not given reference ranges for the blood count, one of the most commonly performed laboratory measurements. Appendix I gives normal values for haematology. Examiners will usually set abnormal results way outside normal limits so that a competent student will spot that they are grossly abnormal without wasting time remembering those awkward details. The core skill of interpreting a full blood count is described on page 174 (Data 5: Blood count).

2. She has a number of symptoms and signs that fit into a coherent picture:
   - Her lack of energy and ankle swelling are caused by the anaemia.
   - Vague upper abdominal pain in an anaemic patient on ibuprofen could be due to a peptic ulcer.
   - It would be worth checking that the pain is truly abdominal and not precipitated by exertion because an old person with such severe anaemia is at risk of angina.
   - The fall might have been mechanical due to the osteoarthritis, or due to syncope associated with her anaemia.

The best response would be not just to offer those interpretations, but to arrange them into a logical sequence of cause and effect: *Her blood film suggests iron deficiency, and that is probably the cause of her lack of energy and ankle swelling. Given that she is on ibuprofen and anaemic, her upper abdominal pain might suggest peptic ulceration, though she is also at risk of angina and I would want to check whether the pain was related to exertion. Her fall may have been mechanical, or syncopal and caused by her anaemia.*

E – *Do you think she should have a blood transfusion?*

It would be easy to be flustered by this question. You probably feel uncertain what to say and attribute your uncertainty to ignorance. In fact, there is no cut-and-dried answer. If ever you are unsure about the best course of action, a reasoned argument will make the best use of what knowledge you have and convey the impression that you are a thoughtful clinician.

The indications for blood transfusion are:

1. Moderate to severe acute blood loss.
2. In the normovolaemic patient:
   - Severe (e.g. Hb < 80 g/l) symptomatic anaemia, particularly if causing cardiovascular compromise.
   - Less severe anaemia if there is a risk that the patient may lose blood acutely.
   - Marrow failure causing symptomatic anaemia; e.g. in a myeloproliferative disease.

The decision to transfuse is quite finely balanced in this case because old people are particularly vulnerable to the complications of anaemia (angina and cerebral ischaemia) but are also particularly prone to left ventricular failure resulting from volume overload. Transfusion would definitely be indicated if Mrs Thomas's fall were due to a gastrointestinal bleed (if, for example, she had malaena on rectal examination). Depending on the severity of her symptoms and her cardiovascular status, there may be an indication for transfusing her even without evidence of acute blood loss.

PROCEDURE SKILLS

E – *How would you minimise the cardiovascular risks of transfusion?*

● Give red cells, rather than whole blood to minimise the volume load.
● Intravenous loop diuretic (e.g. frusemide 20–40 mg) at the start of the transfusion.
● Close observation for signs of volume overload.

When discussing the pros and cons of transfusion, you might comment on Mrs Thomas's relatively normal examination; if the neck veins had been raised or she had basal crackles suggesting left ventricular failure, she would need to be treated with a diuretic before contemplating transfusion for subacute anaemia. Even with a normal cardiovascular examination, you might wish to give intravenous diuretic prophylactically and should certainly observe her carefully for emerging signs of heart failure.

E – *Can you give me the possible complications of blood transfusion, other than the cardiovascular ones?*

Transfusion reaction

● Blood given to the wrong patient
● Reactions due to red cell antibodies other than ABO and anti Rh D
● Non-haemolytic febrile transfusion reactions (e.g. due to white cell antibodies)
● Allergic or anaphylactic reactions.

Metabolic (rare, and usually associated with massive transfusions)

● Hypocalcaemia (caused by the citrate anticoagulant)
● Hyperkalaemia (particularly with older cells which lyse more readily)
● Hypothermia (with large volumes of cold blood).

Infection

Viral

● HIV
● Hepatitis B
● Hepatitis C
● Cytomegalovirus.

Bacterial

● If blood were kept at room temperature long enough for bacterial contamination (hopefully, only a theoretical risk).

E – *You decide to transfuse her; please describe the procedure.*

PROCEDURE SKILLS

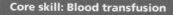

Core skill: Blood transfusion

1. Introduce yourself, explain what you would like to do and obtain consent (Introduction to Procedures; page 187).
   - This should include an explanation of the alternatives to transfusion (see Communication 7: Lumbar puncture).

2. Record in the case notes:
   - The indication for transfusion
   - That the patient consented to transfusion after explanation of the reasons, risks and benefits
   - The name of the person who ordered the blood (legibly).

3. Select the product (whole blood or red cells) and quantity (as a rule of thumb, 1 unit of red cells will raise the plasma haemoglobin by 10 g/l).

4. Order the product in writing (and by telephone in an emergency). The request form should include:
   - Patient's identity number, full name and date of birth
   - Quantity of blood, and when needed
   - Legible signature.

5. Take blood:
   - Check the patient's identity verbally and from her identity bracelet
   - Take 10 ml blood in a tube without anticoagulant
   - Immediately after taking the blood, label the tube with full identification details at the bedside.

6. Ensure that blood reaches the laboratory promptly, where blood will be:
   - Grouped for the ABO and rhesus systems
   - Tested for IgG antibodies that can damage red cells at 37°C
   - Cross-matched; in other words, red cells of an appropriate group will be selected and tested for compatibility with the patient's serum.

7. Prescribe the amount of blood, and duration of the infusion, and arrange for it to be delivered:
   - Blood is stored at 4°C after cross-matching. The infusion must start within 30 min of removing it from the refrigerator, and be completed within 5 h.

8. Check identity:
   - Two people must do this, one a qualified health professional
   - The patient's identity must be checked with the patient herself and against the ID band, lab report and blood bottle
   - The cell type, donation number and expiry date should be checked.

9. Infuse the blood; this must be through a blood administration set, with an integral filter.

10. Observe:
    - Temperature and pulse at time 0, 15 min, 30 min and then hourly

---

Core skill: *(cont'd)*

11. Record details of the transfusion in the case notes:
    - No of units, and their group
    - Any adverse events.
12. Record the transfusion on the patient's fluid chart.

E – *Thirty minutes after starting the transfusion, Mrs Thomas becomes restless and flushed. She develops an urticarial skin rash, headache and abdominal pain. Her temperature is 38°C. What would you do?*

This history is typical of a haemolytic transfusion reaction, which is a medical emergency.

- Stop the transfusion, replace the giving set and keep the line open with 0.9% saline.
- Check her identity against the blood bottle to see if she has received the wrong patient's blood.
- Take blood for:
  - Blood culture
  - FBC, coagulation screen and repeat cross-match
  - Urea and electrolytes.
- Return blood pack and giving set to laboratory.
- Call for senior help.

SUGGESTIONS FOR FURTHER PRACTICE

Ensure that you have been involved closely enough with blood transfusions that you can describe the procedure from experience. Most of this station – particularly the procedure – is a matter of common sense but it will clearly distinguish students who are clinically experienced from those that are not fit to be house officers. The 'core skill' box describes the procedure as defined by the UK blood transfusion authorities, but it would be a hopeless task to try to memorise it at that level of detail. Find a patient who has to have a transfusion and follow the procedure through to familiarise yourself with the steps, then see if you can list the major headings in the box.

PROCEDURE 10 — Finger-prick blood glucose measurement

Level:	*
Setting:	Yourself and the examiner. You are provided with a tray containing dry-wipe, visually-read blood glucose measurement strips[1] and equipment for pricking a finger. A glucose-containing 'artificial blood' solution is provided
Time:	5 min

TASK

E – *Mr Wall, a man in his late 60s, was admitted to your ward with pneumonia last night. His casualty blood glucose level was 12 mmol/l. He has been given no treatment for diabetes. Please show me how you would use the equipment to obtain a blood sample. Use my finger, but talk through the procedure rather than prick it. Please then use this artificial blood solution to show me how to measure blood glucose.*

RESPONSE

Core skill: Finger-prick blood glucose measurement

1. Introduce yourself, explain what you would like to do and obtain consent (Introduction to Procedures; page 187).

2. Ask the patient to wash his hands:
   - To prevent infection (very unlikely)
   - To remove any glucose from the skin.

3. Select from the tray:
   - A strip
   - Several pieces of cotton wool
   - Tissues to place the strip on while wiping it
   - The spring-loaded finger-prick device
   - A lancet
   - A disposable 'platform' for the finger-pricker
   - A stop-watch with second hand (or your own watch).

4. If you are unfamiliar with the strip system, check timing details on the package.[2]

5. Lay the strip with its test surface upwards on a tissue with cotton wool beside it.

6. Position the lancet and platform in the device and 'load' it.

7. Choose a finger/thumb which has not been pricked recently, press finger-pricker firmly against soft part of finger-tip and 'fire'.

---

[1] Depending on hospital policy, visually-read strips or one of various types of meter might be provided.

[2] For the purposes of this description, assume that blood has to be in contact with the test area for 60 s and the result is read 60 s after wiping.

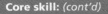

Core skill: *(cont'd)*

8. Hold the finger with the end pointing downwards and massage gently until a drop of blood has formed which is large enough to cover the strip; if insufficient blood, repeat the finger-prick.

9. Bring the strip up to the drop of blood; on contact, blood should cover the entire surface of the test area.

10. After 60 s, wipe.

11. After a further 60 s, compare the test area with the visual check card, decide the result and write it down.

E – *Let us assume that your result was 8.0 mmol/l, what conclusions could you come to?*

You should never try to interpret a blood glucose result without knowing whether or not the patient is fasting. In all but exceptional circumstances, measure glucose only before breakfast or a main meal. In this case, you need to find out if Mr Wall was fasting. As it stands, your answer has to be *'no conclusion'*.

E – *The fasting blood glucose was 8.0 mmol/l. What significance do you attach to that, and what further actions would you take?*

- The result is compatible with a diagnosis of diabetes.[3]
- An abnormal *finger-prick* test result must be confirmed on a *laboratory* measurement before diagnosing diabetes.
- Patients may be transiently hyperglycaemic during an acute illness like pneumonia; you cannot yet conclude that they are permanently diabetic.
- Were the patient definitely diabetic, a fasting blood glucose concentration of 8.0 mmol/l represents moderate, though not 'perfect', glycaemic control. You should ask a dietitian to advise them on a sugar-free diet, notify the general practitioner, and arrange out-patient follow-up.
- A fasting blood glucose measurement (and, possibly, a glucose tolerance test) needs to be repeated when the patient is over the pneumonia.

SUGGESTIONS FOR FURTHER PRACTICE

Any medical student should become competent at glucose measurement early in their clinical training. Since at least 5% of hospital bed-days in the Western world are associated with diabetes, there is no shortage of opportunities. As with all diagnostic procedures, examiners will expect competence in interpreting test results as well as in the procedure itself. Familiarise yourself with the current criteria for diagnosing diabetes.

---

[3] The diagnostic criteria for diabetes are undergoing change at the time of writing. Until now, the WHO criterion for diabetes was > 7.8 mmol/l but a lower level (fasting blood glucose > 7.0 mmol/l) has been adopted in the USA and is likely to become widely accepted.

PROCEDURE SKILLS

PROCEDURE 11	**Aspirate knee joint**
Level:	**
Setting:	**An anatomical model of a knee joint. A trolley with gloves, syringes, needles, antiseptic solution, cotton wool, dressings and specimen tubes is provided. Extension into data interpretation**
Time:	**5 min**

TASK

E – *Please imagine that this is the knee of a patient with a painful, swollen joint. You have found a large effusion and decide to perform a diagnostic aspiration. Please demonstrate the technique.*

RESPONSE

Core skill: Knee joint aspiration

1. Introduce yourself, explain what you would like to do and obtain consent (Introduction to Procedures; page 187).

2. Position the knee slightly flexed and supported by a pillow.

3. Examine the knee to define the normal anatomy and confirm the presence of an effusion.

4. Wash your hands and put on gloves.

5. Clean the skin over the entry site (see below).

6. Attach a green (21 G) needle to a 5 or 10 ml syringe.

7. Press gently on the medial aspect of the patella with your free hand to displace fluid laterally and open up the gap between the patella and femur.

8. Introduce the needle from the upper, lateral aspect of the patello-femoral joint aiming medially and downwards, aspirating as you go.

9. Withdraw 5–10 ml fluid.

10. Withdraw the needle and syringe, press firmly with cotton wool until any bleeding has stopped and apply a dressing.

E – *The fluid looks turbid. Numerous white cells are seen on microscopy and Gram-positive cocci are seen on Gram stain. What action would you take?*

Any acute monoarthritis is a medical emergency. In this case, the diagnosis is septic arthritis. Management consists of:

- An intravenous antibiotic; this is likely to be a staphylococcal infection so flucloxacillin is an appropriate choice.
- Repeated aspiration of the joint or arthroscopy and joint washout to prevent cartilage destruction.
- Bed rest to take weight off the joint.
- Analgesia.

See the core skill box for the interpretation of joint aspirates.

Core skill: Interpretation of joint aspirate

Colour

- **Clear** fluid suggests a non-inflammatory effusion.
- **Turbid** fluid suggests an inflammatory process; it may also be blood-stained.
- **Milky** fluid may occur in crystal arthritis.
- Heavy **blood-staining** may indicate a haemarthrosis.

Microscopy

- **White count:** very low in a non-inflammatory effusion; extremely high in septic arthritis.
- **Gram staining** for bacterial infection.
- With **polarised light** to diagnose crystal synovitis (gout or pseudogout).

Culture

- For **bacterial infection**.
- For **tuberculosis**, if clinically indicated.

SUGGESTIONS FOR FURTHER PRACTICE

You may not have aspirated a joint on a patient by the time of qualification but you MUST have observed the procedure (and, ideally, aspiration of other joints as well) and you should practise on an anatomical model if one is available.

PROCEDURE SKILLS

PROCEDURE 12 **Basic life support**

Level:	*
Setting:	Resuscitation mannequin
Time:	5 min

TASK

E – *You and a friend are walking along the street when you find this man lying half on the road and half on the pavement. Please show me what you would do.*

RESPONSE

There is no clinical skill more clearly defined than basic life support. You are likely to be marked very harshly (probably failed outright) if you cannot manage at least a competent demonstration of this skill.

Initial assessment

Ensure your own safety and that of the victim; tell the examiner that you would move the person to safety.

Gently shake the victim's shoulders and ask loudly *are you all right*?

E – *The person does not respond.*

Shout for help.

Airway maintenance

Place your hand on his forehead and gently tilt his head back, keeping your thumb and index finger free to close his nose if rescue breathing is required.

With your fingertips under the point of the victim's chin, lift the chin to open the airway.

Check breathing

Keeping the airway open, look, listen and feel for breathing for 10 s:

- Look for chest movements
- Listen at the victim's mouth for breath sounds
- Feel for air on your cheek.

Send your friend to get help.

Expired air ventilation (rescue breathing)

Remove any visible obstructions from the victim's mouth, including dislodged dentures, but leave well-fitting dentures in place.

Give two **effective** rescue breaths, each of which makes the chest rise and fall:

- Ensure head tilt and chin lift
- Pinch the soft part of his nose closed with the index finger and thumb of your hand on his forehead
- Open his mouth a little, but maintain chin lift
- Blow steadily into his mouth for 1.5–2.0 s, watching for his chest to rise as in normal breathing
- Maintaining head tilt and chin lift, take your mouth away from the victim and watch for his chest to fall as air comes out
- Repeat this sequence for the second breath.

Check circulation

Assess the victim for signs of a circulation, taking no more than 10 s:

- Look for any movement, including swallowing or breathing
- Check the carotid pulse.

Chest compression

Assuming you can find no signs of a circulation, start chest compression:

- Place one hand on top of the other, with the fingers interlocked and the heel of the lower hand over the middle of the lower half of the sternum.
- Position yourself vertically above the victim's chest and, with your arms straight, press down on the sternum to depress it 4–5 cm. Be sure that your fingers do not press on the ribs.
- Release the pressure, without losing contact between the hand and the sternum, then repeat at a rate of about 100 times a minute; compression and release should take an equal amount of time.

Combine rescue breathing and compression:

- After 15 compressions, tilt the head, lift the chin and give 2 effective breaths
- Return your hands without delay to the correct position on the sternum; continue compressions and breaths in a ratio of 15 to 2.

When your friend returns from summoning help, he should take over chest compression and work on the opposite side of the victim from you. You should use a ratio of 5 to 1; chest compression must cease during inflation.

How long to continue

Until:

- Help arrives

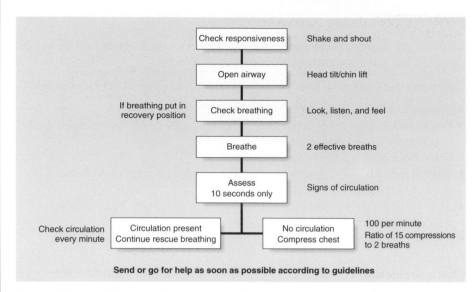

Figure 6.5 Core skill: basic life support. This figure is reproduced with the kind permission of the publishers from Br Med J (1998) 316: 1870–1876

- The victim shows signs of life
- You become exhausted.

E – *How would you have acted differently if you had been on your own when you found the patient collapsed?*

If an adult is found collapsed, it should be assumed that he has a heart problem. The quicker a defibrillator arrives, the better the outcome so it is recommended that a lone rescuer should call for an ambulance before starting resuscitation **unless** the problem is trauma or drowning, in which case a lone rescuer should perform resuscitation for about 1 min before going to call for help.

It would show awareness of the current resuscitation guidelines to say what you would do if you were on your own without waiting for the examiner to prompt you.

SUGGESTIONS FOR FURTHER PRACTICE

Practise with a mannequin until you are completely confident in the procedure. The marking criteria are so clearly laid down that you should have no difficulty role-playing this station with a friend. Arrange to be an observer on a hospital cardiac arrest team so that you can gain real confidence by putting the skill into practice 'in anger'. Do not be satisfied just with learning basic life support; move on to advanced life support (Procedure 3).

PROCEDURE 13 Venepuncture

Level:	*
Setting:	An anatomical arm, venepuncture tray, sharps bin and vacuum venepuncture system
Time:	5 min

TASK

E – *Please obtain 5 ml of heparinised blood. Speak to me as though I were the subject having the venepuncture.*

RESPONSE

Hospitals usually have written policies for common procedures like venepuncture; although there is little scope for variation, you should follow the local policy. Some simple points are:

- There is no evidence that cleaning the skin with an alcohol swab reduces the risk of infection or contamination in a 'socially clean' arm.
- Bending the arm over a cotton wool swab causes more bruising than pressure over the vein with a finger.
- Resheathing increases the risk of needlestick injuries.

Communication aspects of the skill are covered in the introductory section, page 187.

Core skill: Venepuncture

1. Introduce yourself, explain what you would like to do and obtain consent (Introduction to Procedures; page 187).

2. Select equipment from the tray:
   - Needle and hub
   - Heparin tube
   - Cotton wool
   - Cuff
   - Gloves.

3. Position the arm and identify a vein.

4. Explain what you plan to do and check that the patient is willing for you to proceed.

5. Apply the cuff and re-check the vein.

6. Put on gloves.

7. Explain to the patient what they will feel.

PROCEDURE SKILLS

227

Core skill: *(cont'd)*

8. Attach a needle to the needle-holder.

9. Insert a tube into the needle-holder.

10. Insert the needle into the vein, bevel upwards.

11. Loosen the cuff once blood appears in the tube.

12. Pick up a ball of cotton wool.

13. When the tube is full, withdraw it from the needle-holder.

14. Withdraw the needle and press cotton wool over the exit site.

15. Ask the patient to press on the cotton wool without bending their arm.

16. Discard the needle without re-sheathing.

17. Rock the tube.

18. Remove the gloves.

19. Check how the patient feels and thank them.

Even if you are not asked to label the tube, show the examiner that you would now do so; include the patient's first and last name, hospital number and date of birth.

The examiner might ask you about:

- Swabbing the skin; you could volunteer: *I would not use an alcohol swab, provided the skin was 'socially clean'.*
- Safe techniques for needle disposal.
- Health and safety practices.
- How the anticoagulants in the tube work, or which tube is used for which test.

SUGGESTIONS FOR FURTHER PRACTICE

Do not approach even the most elementary OSCE without being absolutely familiar with the process of venepuncture. You should be able to do it fluently both on an anatomical arm and on a volunteer. You should have done the procedure enough times not to fumble with the equipment and be able to obtain blood easily from all but the hardest veins. Find out the policy for venepuncture in your hospital. Be clear about the health hazards associated with handling sharps. Know which anticoagulant is in which coloured tube, how the anticoagulants work and which tube is needed for which test in your hospital.

PROCEDURE SKILLS

PROCEDURE 14 | Suture skin

Level:	**
Setting:	A pad of simulated skin with a 2 cm cut. A trolley, sterile pack, gloves, syringes, needles and vials of local anaesthetic are provided
Time:	5 min

TASK

E – *Please imagine that this is the skin of a patient's arm. Please suture the skin wound under local anaesthetic. I will act as your assistant. The surface of this trolley has been cleaned; you can use it for your sterile pack. Let us imagine that the patient is unconscious and that you have consent to do the procedure.*

RESPONSE

Core skill: Skin suturing

1. Wash your hands.

2. Ask your assistant to open the sterile pack and put the inner pack onto the trolley.

3. Open the inner pack.

4. Ask your assistant to open the pack of sterile gloves and drop them onto the sterile field.

5. Dry your hands on the sterile towel and put on the gloves.

6. Ask your assistant to pour antiseptic solution into the receiver.

7. Request a 5 ml syringe, 21 G needle to draw up anaesthetic, and a 25 G needle to infiltrate.

8. Request a suture; e.g. a 4/0 synthetic, non-absorbable monofilament, with a curved needle.

9. Ask your assistant to open the vial of anaesthetic; e.g. lignocaine with 1/200 000 adrenaline (to minimise bleeding). Attach a 21 G needle to the syringe and draw up 5 ml of anaesthetic. Detach the needle without resheathing, discard it and attach a 25 G needle.

10. Clean the skin with antiseptic-soaked cotton wool, held with forceps.

11. Infiltrate the skin with local anaesthetic, drawing back on the syringe before injecting.

12. When the anaesthetic has had time to work, grasp a curved needle with needle-holding forceps.

13. Pick up a skin edge with toothed forceps.

Core skill: *(cont'd)*

14. Pass the needle perpendicularly through the skin 1–2 mm away from the wound edge and into the wound just below the dermis. Grasp the point of the needle and pull it and a length of suture through the needle-hole.

15. Pass the needle through the opposite skin edge and upwards through the skin.

16. Tighten and appose the skin edges, without tension and with slight eversion of the edges.

17. Knot around suture-holding forceps.

18. Repeat, with sutures 5–10 mm apart.

E – *How soon can you start suturing after the anaesthetic?*

It may take 5–10 min for the anaesthetic to take effect. You should check that the patient cannot feel a sharp needle applied to the skin before proceeding.

E – *When should the sutures be removed?*

After about 7 days. Scalp wounds heal faster so sutures can be removed earlier.

E – *What are the possible side-effects of the anaesthetic?*

- Adrenaline can cause ischaemic tissue necrosis; it is safe to use it on the skin of the trunk or a limb, but it should never be used on an extremity (e.g. finger, ear lobe, nose).
- A massive dose of intravenous lignocaine inadvertently given intravenously could, theoretically, cause convulsions, depression of the central nervous system, heart block or acute heart failure. That is why you must draw back on the syringe before infiltrating to ensure that the drug is not given intravenously.

E – *Under what circumstances should a tetanus immunisation be given?*

- If patient has not received a 'booster' dose within the previous 10 years.
- If the wound is contaminated.

SUGGESTIONS FOR FURTHER PRACTICE

Skin suturing is a core clinical skill, without which you cannot perform more advanced procedures such as insertion of a chest drain. Lifelike skin pads will be available for practice if your medical school has a well-equipped clinical skills laboratory. You should be experienced at performing the skill on patients; there is no shortage of opportunities in casualty departments. You will be penalised heavily if you are incompetent at suturing by the time you have reached intermediate or senior level.

PROCEDURE 15 | Arterial blood sampling

Level:	***
Setting:	An anatomical arm; extension into data interpretation
Time:	5 min

TASK

E – *Please imagine that this arm belongs to a patient with renal failure who is extremely short of breath. I would like you to take arterial blood for blood gas analysis. You have a tray with all relevant equipment available to you.*

RESPONSE

The examiner is testing the core skill of arterial puncture. Since you have been offered an anatomical arm, your choice is between the radial and brachial arteries. The description that follows applies to the radial artery, but the brachial and femoral are little different. Do not forget the communication and ethical aspects discussed in the introduction to this chapter, page 187, and elaborated under Procedure 13: Venepuncture.

Core skill: Radial arterial puncture

1. Introduce yourself, explain the procedure and ask for the patient's consent (Introduction to Procedures: Page 187).

2. Select equipment from the tray:
   - 23 G (blue) needles, 2 ml syringe and cap for syringe
   - Heparin
   - Cotton wool.

3. Attach needle, draw a little heparin into syringe, expel and discard needle.

4. Attach fresh needle.

5. Explain and check that patient is willing for you to proceed.

6. Position arm with wrist extended.

7. Locate artery with index and middle fingers of non-dominant hand.

8. Explain to the patient what they will feel.

9. Insert needle at 30° to skin at point of maximum pulsation.

10. Advance until arterial blood flushes back into syringe.

11. Allow arterial pressure to drive about 2 ml blood into the syringe; aspirate gently if needed.

Core skill: *(cont'd)*

12. Pick up cotton wool with non-dominant hand.

13. Withdraw needle/syringe assembly and press firmly over puncture site with cotton wool.

14. Press for 5 min.

15. Remove and discard needle.

16. Cap syringe.

E – *This is the result of the test. The reference ranges are shown in brackets. How do you interpret the test?*

pO_2 (kPa)	pCO_2 (kPa)	pH	Bicarbonate (mmol/l)
27*	2.5**	6.9	8
(12–15)	(4.5–6.0)	(7.38–7.42)	(24–30)
	*200 mmHg	**19 mmHg	

Never attempt to interpret blood gas results without knowing whether they were taken on room air or on oxygen; if on oxygen, what was the concentration? In this case, the pO_2 is so high that it could only be explained by the patient being on oxygen therapy. The examiner will give you credit for asking, particularly if you phrase your question: *The pO_2 is very high. I suspect that the patient is receiving oxygen therapy. May I ask what concentration?*

What is clearly abnormal is the patient's acid-base status. You might reason your way through these results as follows:

● The low pH shows that the patient is acidotic.
● The low bicarbonate shows that it is a **metabolic** acidosis
● The low pCO_2 is compensatory; the patient is 'blowing off' CO_2 because of the metabolic acidosis and that is why he is breathless.

E – *What further test would you do?*

The one further test to characterise the metabolic acidosis is to measure serum chloride, from which you can measure the anion gap. The examiner has said that the patient has renal failure, which can cause acidosis by impairing hydrogen ion excretion. As pH and bicarbonate fall, serum chloride rises to maintain electrical neutrality such that the anion gap $((Na^+ + K^+) - (Cl^- + HCO_3^-))$ is less than

10 mmol/l. The value of calculating the anion gap is to distinguish that situation from an acidosis caused by accumulation of lactic acid (lactic acidosis), ketoacids (as in diabetic ketoacidosis) or poisoning with e.g. salicylate or ethylene glycol. In these situations there is no compensatory rise in chloride and the anion gap exceeds 10 mmol/l.

The core skill box shows the pattern of pCO_2, pH and bicarbonate in respiratory and metabolic acidosis and alkalosis, the four basic acid/base abnormalities that you must be able to recognise. Interpreting blood gases is a core clinical skill, as described in the box. If you are rusty on the underlying principles, you need to brush up your knowledge of acid/base biochemistry.

Core skill: Interpreting blood gas measurements

1. Be sure that you know the inspired oxygen concentration.

2. Look at the pO_2 and pCO_2; is there respiratory disease?
   Hypoxia with a low pCO_2 signifies ventilation perfusion mismatching, or type 1 respiratory failure.
   Hypoxia with a raised pCO_2 have ventilatory failure, or type 2 respiratory failure.

3. Scan the pH and bicarbonate; is there an acid/base disorder?
   If **acidotic:**   A low bicarbonate shows that it is a metabolic acidosis
                      A high pCO_2 indicates a respiratory acidosis
   If **alkalotic:** A high bicarbonate shows that it is a metabolic akalosis
                      A low pCO_2 signifies a respiratory alkalosis

4. If there is a metabolic acidosis, measure chloride:

	Metabolic acidosis	Respiratory acidosis	Respiratory alkalosis	Metabolic alkalosis
pH	↓	↓	↑	↑
pCO_2	(↓)	↑	↓	(↑)
Bicarbonate	↓	(↑)	(↓)	↑

↓, fall; ↑, increase; ( ) compensatory as opposed to primary change.

Both arterial blood sampling and blood gas interpretation are such basic clinical skills that you should expect the two to be coupled together. A strong candidate would not just interpret the blood gases but link them to the cue about renal failure and extend into the anion gap without being prompted.

SUGGESTIONS FOR FURTHER PRACTICE

Seize every opportunity to practise blood gas sampling. It is done many times

PROCEDURE SKILLS

each day in any emergency medicine department. Although patients in intensive care units usually have indwelling arterial lines and are unavailable for you to practise the sampling procedure, they provide abundant opportunities to interpret the results. Do not attempt to do so until you have mastered the principles and can draw the table in the box from first principles. Learn the reference ranges by interpreting blood gas results 'blind' until the limits of normal become second nature.

PROCEDURE 16	**Death certification**
Level:	***
Setting:	A written exercise
Time:	10 min

TASK

The examiner hands you a card that reads as follows:

> You are a house officer at St Elsewhere's Hospital. Mr Kenneth Sidebotham, a diabetic patient aged 68, was admitted under your care on 16 May 1998. Before admission, he was virtually housebound due to emphysema. He had a coronary artery bypass graft 8 years ago. Three years ago, he had coronary angiography for unstable angina which showed advanced coronary artery disease that was not amenable to surgery. His admission on this occasion was with severe cardiac chest pain. His ECG showed an anterior infarct and he had a massive enzyme rise. You reviewed him before going off duty last night, and found him to be hypotensive and in severe left ventricular failure. This morning (19 May) you came on duty to be told by a fellow house officer that she was called to certify Mr Sidebotham dead only an hour later.

E – *Please write a death certificate for Mr Sidebotham. His widow has not been approached for permission for a post-mortem but is coming into the hospital later to collect the certificate.*

RESPONSE

The cause of death is straightforward and you are in a position to complete the certificate because:

- You saw Mr Sidebotham within 14 days of death.
- Although you did not see the patient after death, another practitioner did.

Figure 6.6 shows an example of how you might complete the certificate and the process is described in the Core Skill Box on page 237.

E – *After you have written the death certificate, you meet Mrs Sidebotham and give her your condolences. She tells you that her husband had been a coal miner and had received a pension for the last 15 years because he had pneumoconiosis. What are the implications of this information?*

The death should be referred to the Coroner because Mr Sidebotham had an

Name of deceased: _Kenneth Sidebotham_

Date of death as stated to me: _18TH_ day of _May 1998_. Age as stated to me: _68_

Place of death: _St. Elsewhere's Hospital_

Last seen alive by me: _18TH_ day of _May 1998_

1	The certified cause of death takes account of information obtained from post-mortem.
(2)	Information from post-mortem may be available later.
3	Post-mortem not being held.
4	I have reported this death to the Coroner for further action.

a)	Seen after death by me.
(b)	Seen after death by another medical practitioner but not by me.
c)	Not seen after death by a medical practitioner.

CAUSE OF DEATH

The condition thought to be the Underlying Cause of Death should appear in the lowest completed line of Part 1.

I (a)   Disease or condition directly leading to death .... _Myocardial infarct_

  (b)   Other disease or condition, if any, leading to I(a) .... _Coronary atherosclerosis_

  (c)   Other disease or condition, if any, leading to I(b) .... _Diabetes mellitus_

II   Other significant conditions CONTRIBUTING TO THE DEATH but .... _Chronic emphysema_ not related to the disease or condition causing it.

Approximate interval between onset and death

Two days ....

Figure 6.6 Completed death certificate.

PROCEDURE SKILLS

industrial disease. If you do not do so, the Registrar will reject the death certificate. Although this seems an added complication at such a delicate moment, you will save Mrs Sidebotham extra distress and inconvenience by explaining that to her now and withdrawing the death certificate that you have just written.

E – *What are the indications for referring a death to the coroner?*

The answer to this question is given in the Core Skill Box on page 237.

E – *What would you do if you were unsure whether to refer a case to the Coroner?*

• Ring the Coroner's office for advice.

Core skill: Completing a death certificate

When it comes to completing the cause of death:

- I(a) must show the disease which actually caused death – in this case a myocardial infarct – not the **mode of death**, in this case heart failure. Generally speaking, any diagnosis which includes the word 'failure' will lead the registrar to refer the case to the Coroner, causing potential delay and distress to the family.

- Any disease(s) that led to death should be entered in a logical sequence. Go over it in your mind and it should read: "I(a) was caused by I(b) which was caused by I(c)". Go over it in reverse order and it should read: "I(c) led to I(b) which led to I(a)".

Do:

- Write clearly.

- Complete the certificate as fully and accurately as possible.

Do not:

- Use abbreviations.

- Use question marks or vague terms such as 'probable'.

- Give 'old age' as the cause of death unless (a) you are unable to be more specific and (b) the patient was aged 70 or over.

- Complete a certificate if there are grounds to report the case to the Coroner (see below).

Core skill: Choosing which patients to refer to the coroner

1. Cause of death unknown.

2. Deceased not seen by certifying doctor either after death or within the 14 days before death.

3. Death violent, unnatural or suspicious.

4. Death may have been due to:
   - An accident
   - Neglect (by self or other(s))
   - Industrial disease
   - An abortion
   - Suicide.

5. Death occurred during an operation or before recovery from anaesthetic.

6. Death occurred during or shortly after detention in prison or police custody.

SUGGESTIONS FOR FURTHER PRACTICE

As a senior student, accompany your house officer (or general practitioner) when they write death certificates. Decide what you would write on the certificates of patients that you have been involved with. Make your own mind up when one of them dies whether or not the case should be referred to the Coroner. If in doubt, consult a histopathologist, who will be very expert on the regulations.

CHAPTER 7

Communication skills

Introduction

Good communication is central to clinical competence and it is likely to have a prominent place in OSCE examinations. This section covers some situations that demand very specific communication skills, and in which your competence as a communicator will be the central point of the assessment. However, communication skills cannot be tested in isolation. They take you to some of the most sensitive and difficult issues that may arise in medical life such as your attitudes towards patients, your awareness of ethical issues, and medical knowledge as diverse as the nitty-gritty of hypertension (Communication 6) and the practicalities of Ramadan in an Asian person with diabetes (Communication 10). This section should be read in conjunction with Chapter 8, Attitudes, which introduces a number of closely related issues in the general area of ethics and professional values.

Communication skills are not restricted to this section. You are shown elsewhere in the book how you might be assessed on your ability to communicate:

- With a patient, when taking a history, examining, or performing a procedure. See, for example, Chapter 6, Procedures, in which every core skill starts with communication.
- With the examiner, when interpreting data or discussing attitudinal issues. See, for example, Attitudes 1.

WHAT ARE COMMUNICATION SKILLS?

Although this book describes a number of individual skills, you will see that there are relatively straightforward principles underpinning them. With experience, you will become adept at applying them to specific situations. For example, the principles of handling emotionally charged situations described in detail under Communication 8: Break bad news, can be summarised as follows:

- Set up the room appropriately.
- Use verbal and non-verbal techniques to make it easy for the patient to express themself.
- Wherever possible, ASK the patient rather than TELL them; help them feel in control of the interview.
- Respond to the patient's emotions and put them into words.
- Explore what makes the patient experience those emotions.
- Clarify the facts; use simple language and don't rush.
- Inform and educate.
- Where there is conflict, try to see the patient's point of view and always respect their autonomy.
- Offer any help you can, including a further consultation.
- Summarise, thank and close.

THE STATIONS

The content of this section falls into four main categories. Some stations cover more than one.

Explaining

- Explain 24-h urine collection: Communication 6
- Teach inhaler technique: Communication 3
- Explain statin therapy: Communication 1.

Obtaining consent

- Explain statin therapy: Communication 1
- Endoscopy: Communication 5
- Lumbar puncture: Communication 7
- Discuss HIV testing: Communication 12.

Communication with third parties

- Discuss with a carer: Communication 4
- Cross-cultural communication: Communication 10.

Difficult and emotionally-charged situations

- Respond to a patient's distress: Communication 11
- Break bad news: Communications 8 and 13
- Respond to a patient's dissatisfaction: Communication 9
- Discuss a 'Do not resuscitate' order: Communication 2
- Discuss with a carer: Communication 4
- Cross-cultural communication: Communication 10.

See also: History 6: Erectile dysfunction, for a discussion of how to broach a sensitive topic; History 8: Collapse, for how to respond to a talkative patient; History 1: Chest pain, for an illustration of good listening skills; and History 7: Headache, for an illustration of poor listening skills.

HOW TO REVISE FOR COMMUNICATION STATIONS

Not all medical schools will give you the luxury of standardised patients and video-feedback on your skills so your ability as a communicator might not be put to the test until the OSCE examination. With forethought, that situation need never arise. Each station ends with some suggestions as to how you could develop your communication skills. You can work with one or more fellow students and critique each others' performance using the criteria listed in the individual stations. If, having practised, you are still unsure about the skills or the terminology used in describing them, then it is time to enlist help from a teacher. Please regard the dialogues in this book as illustrative. Do not attempt to adopt them verbatim. Understand the principles that lie behind them, observe skilled communicators at work and develop your own style of communication.

USEFUL RESOURCES

An excellent, short text of communication skills:

Lloyd M, Bor R (1996) Communication Skills for Medicine. Edinburgh: Churchill Livingstone

A CD set which describes communication skills and illustrates them with short video clips:

Buckman R, Korsch B, Baile W. A practical guide to communication skills in clinical practice. Medical Audio Visual Communications Inc. Contact the publisher at: http://www.mavc.com

COMMUNICATION 1	**Explain statin therapy**
Level:	***
Setting:	Standardised patient sitting in an interview room with a desk
Time:	10 min

TASK

E – *Mr Wells, who you are going to interview in a moment, has had the misfortune of having an anterior myocardial infarct at the age of 55. He made an uneventful recovery from the heart attack and is taking aspirin, atenolol and lisinopril. He received healthy-living advice when he left hospital but is not on any lipid-lowering treatment. It is now 3 months after the heart attack and he is back at work as a warehouseman. Put yourself in the position of a house officer working in general practice. You have received his blood lipid results, which are as follows:*

Mr John Wells.　　Age 55.

Plasma cholesterol 6.9 mmol/l
LDL-cholesterol 4.7 mmol/l
HDL-cholesterol 1.1 mmol/l
Triglycerides 1.2 mmol/l

Comment: Increased cardiovascular risk. Consider statin therapy.

E – *This is a difficult station and you have up to 5 minutes to read those results and another document which I am about to give you. This is a short abstract summarising some of the results of the 4S, or Scandinavian Simvastatin Survival Study.*

Patients aged 35–70 years with angina or acute myocardial infarction who had serum cholesterol levels of 5.5–8.0 despite diet treatment, and serum triglyceride levels below 2.6 mmol/l, were randomised to receive simvastatin or placebo for a median of 5.4 years.

Mortality in patients on simvastatin was 8.2% compared with 11.5% in patients on placebo. The absolute reduction in risk was 3.3% (95% CI 1.6–5.1%; $P < 0.001$); number needed to treat (NNT) 30 (95% CI 20–64).

There were fewer coronary events in patients on simvastatin (15.9% vs 22.6%; $P < 0.001$; NNT 15; CI 11–23).

E – *Mr Wells does not know his cholesterol result but has come to surgery for it. Please demonstrate to me in about 5 minutes how you would broach the result and any action you might take on it.*

RESPONSE

This complex station covers the following:

- Knowledge of hyperlipidaemia and coronary prevention
- The ability to read and understand clinical trial results
- Communication, including:
  - Explanation
  - Reaching agreement about treatment
- Knowledge of statins.

The commentary follows those headings. The core skill box pulls them together into a sequence which you could role-play with a class-mate.

It would be easy to be 'phased' by the way this station is set up but there is a generous allocation of time and the brief given by the examiner contains much of the information needed to interview Mr Wells. You may have been thrown by not being given reference values for the plasma lipids but all the information you needed was in the abstract. Any student who had never looked at a set of lipid results and had not developed expertise at reading clinical trial results would flounder. However:

- Cardiovascular disease is the major treatable cause of death in the Western world.
- Doctors are required to practice 'evidence-based medicine', which is impossible if you cannot read the evidence (Sackett et al, 1997).

So you would be well advised to approach final exams well prepared for these topics.

Hyperlipidaemia and coronary prevention

The major risk factors for ischaemic heart disease (IHD) are smoking, hypertension and hyperlipidaemia. Other important ones are diabetes and a family history of IHD. The benefits of lipid-lowering are greatest for patients who, like Mr Wells, have had a heart attack. You should establish which other risk factors he has, although the plasma cholesterol result, coupled with the results of the 4S study, show you that he is hyperlipidaemic and would benefit from simvastatin therapy.

It is always good practice when taking or presenting histories to show your awareness of risk factors for disease. In the case of IHD, that is essential because correcting each of those risk factors is proven to prevent heart attacks and the presence of any one risk factor increases the need to treat the others. You should ask him about diabetes, family history and smoking, and volunteer to the examiner at the end of the interview that you would like to measure his blood pressure.

Interpreting clinical trials

Points you should consider when applying clinical trial results to your patient are:

- Is your patient comparable to the patients in the trial? Mr Wells certainly is.
- How good is the trial? You have been spared that question in this case, but you would be well advised to be able to answer questions on 'critical appraisal' of clinical trials.
- How strong is the evidence? In this case, one life will be saved and two coronary events prevented for every 30 patients treated with simvastatin for 5 years.
- How do those results fit with the patient's personal needs and preferences? That will be covered under 'Communication'.

One of the most important things that evidence-based medicine has taught us is a clear way to present clinical trial results. However, the abstract above contains some abbreviations with which you may not be familiar. Every medical student should know what a *p*-value is, but how many are so comfortable with confidence intervals that they could include them in their conversation with a patient? If Mr Wells showed a keen interest in the likely benefits of his simvastatin prescription, you could show the examiner how well you understand the abstract by saying: *We can be 95% sure that at least 1 life will be saved for every 64 people treated with simvastatin for 5 years, and the figure could be as high as 1 in 20.* If you are in any doubt about the following, look them up in a basic textbook of clinical epidemiology or evidence-based medicine (see the reference):

- Absolute risk reduction (ARR)
- Relative risk reduction (RRR)
- Number needed to treat (NNT)
- 95% confidence interval (CI)
- *p* value
- Standard deviation and standard error.

Communication

Doctors are so free with prescriptions that you may not have seen the relevance of 'informed consent' to this case. The core skill of obtaining informed consent is covered in Communication 7: Lumbar puncture. The patient is free not to take a prescribed drug, and the high rate of 'non-compliance' with prescribed drugs shows just how many people exercise that freedom. The process of consent may be verbal and relatively informal but it demands a good explanation; the core skill of giving an explanation is covered in Communication 6: Explain 24-h urine collection. Your interview should use all the communication skills described in those and other stations as described in the Core Skill Box on page 246.

Statin therapy

The examiner will expect you to know about this commonly prescribed class of drugs in terms of:

> ## Core skill: Reaching agreement about treatment
>
> 1. Introduce yourself and establish a rapport.
>
> 2. Explain the reason to consider treatment (in this case, the fact that the cholesterol level increases the risk of future heart attacks).
>
> 3. Give the patient a chance to react to that information.
>
> 4. Explain the likely benefits of therapy as precisely as possible.
>
> 5. Explain what treatment will mean to the patient, e.g. frequency of dosing and duration of therapy (at least 5 years and probably indefinite in this case).
>
> 6. Explain the possible side-effects and how they weigh up against the likely benefits.
>
> 7. Give ample opportunities for the patient to react to the information, ask questions and add new information.
>
> 8. Ask whether the patient would like to proceed with therapy.
>
> 9. Allow the patient time to consider the choice and seek further information, if necessary.

Pharmacology:

- Competitive inhibitors of HMG CoA reductase, an enzyme involved in cholesterol synthesis.
- The main effect is to reduce total and LDL cholesterol; some statins also lower triglycerides significantly.

Practicalities

- Once-daily dosing, usually taken at night.

Benefits

- Reduction of cardiovascular risk, as discussed above. Statins also:
  - Cause regression of coronary atheromatous plaques
  - May ameliorate peripheral vascular as well as coronary artery disease
  - Slightly reduce the risk of stroke.

Side-effects

- **Major** – both rare:
  - Hepatocellular damage
  - Myalgia/myositis.
- **Minor**
  - Headache, minor increase in liver enzymes, abdominal pain, nausea and vomiting.

SUGGESTIONS FOR FURTHER PRACTICE

You must be knowledgeable and experienced in the primary and secondary prevention of ischaemic heart disease. Take every opportunity to observe and be involved in it. Many of the communication issues in this station are 'generic' but the approach to negotiating drug therapy (achieving 'concordance' with your patient) is a specific skill. Finally, you must develop your skill at reading clinical trials. Find a major recent trial and try calculating the absolute and relative risk reductions and number needed to treat.

REFERENCE

Sackett DL, Richardson WS, Rosenberg W, Haynes RB 1997 Evidence-based Medicine. How to Practice and Teach EBM. Churchill Livingstone: Edinburgh

COMMUNICATION SKILLS

COMMUNICATION 2 | Discuss a 'do not resuscitate' order

Level:	***
Setting:	The examiner interviews you across a desk
Time:	10 min

TASK

E – *You are the house officer on a medical ward. You call into the ward and the nursing staff are having coffee in the office. One of them asks: 'Mr Taylor's just been readmitted. Is he for resuscitation?' You know that he is 72 and has heart failure. He was discharged 3 days ago after 6 weeks on the ward. He was discharged on large doses of tablets and you were not optimistic that he would cope. He is not well supported by family, rarely leaves the house, and depends on a home help to do the shopping. He became depressed during his last admission. How would you answer the nurse?*

RESPONSE

This question is about a 'Do not resuscitate' order but note the way the examiner posed the question. Was the detail about the nurses having coffee irrelevant? You are being tested on your attitude towards teamworking. The nurse, like you, knows Mr Taylor and should contribute to the decision. You should ask her opinion and handle the decision jointly. In doing so, you are not just practising good teamwork but upholding good, ethical practice within the team. A good response to the nurse's question would be to ask *What do you think?* and *Have you discussed it with Mr Taylor?*

Resuscitation status

'Do not resuscitate' orders may be made without consulting the patient if:

- There is no likelihood that resuscitation will be successful.
- The patient's quality of life is extremely poor.
- The patient is not able to make the decision, i.e. comatose or not mentally competent.

In all other circumstances, the patient must be involved in the decision himself. The patient's family may also be involved if he is unable to speak for himself or wishes them to be, but remember that your first duty is to him. You have been given no evidence that Mr Taylor is mentally incompetent. You have insufficient evidence that resuscitation would be futile or that his quality of life is too poor to justify resuscitation to make an independent decision; however, there is real doubt that resuscitation would be in his interests. Having exchanged views with the nursing staff, the decision must be discussed with Mr Taylor.

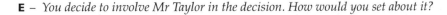

E – *You decide to involve Mr Taylor in the decision. How would you set about it?*

Just as the views of the nursing staff were as important as your own in airing the issues surrounding his resuscitation status, the involvement of the nurse who is closest to him is equally important in helping Mr Taylor arrive at a decision. Now the emphasis of this station shifts from your **knowledge of ethics** and **attitude towards multiprofessional working** to **communication skills**.

Communication issues

The format of the discussion should have many similarities with the 'breaking bad news' interview (Communications 8 and 13).

Setting

- Privacy: a quiet office with comfortable chairs is better than the bedside in an open ward.
- Lack of interruptions: leave your bleep with a colleague and redirect the phone.
- Pacing: allow yourself enough time to conduct the interview in an unhurried way.

Opening

- Invitation: invite Mr Taylor into the room yourself, and ensure that he is comfortable.

E – *I would like you to role play the interview. I am now Mr Taylor. Use your own name, but call yourself 'Dr'. Imagine that you are accompanied by Jane, the staff nurse.*

S – *Mr Taylor, you and I got to know one another during your last admission. I am Dr Smith. You know staff nurse and I think you are on first name terms with her. How would you like me to address you?*

P – Call me Jim.

Listening skills

- Pay attention to your verbal and non-verbal listening skills throughout the interview.

Introduce the subject

- Warning shot: it is good practice to build up towards the main point of your interview. You might do this by saying: *I have something important to discuss with you.*
- Respond to emotions: you must balance the **factual** and **emotional** content of the discussion. As the interview proceeds and Mr Taylor responds, it is good practice to concentrate on **emotions before facts**, by saying, for example: *I can see that you are distressed by this discussion.*

- Empathy: he may find it supportive if you show that you share some of his emotions, for example: *Knowing you as well as I do, I find it hard to confront you with such painful facts.*

Arrive at a decision

- Narrative approach: you may find it easiest to bring Mr Taylor to the point of the decision by giving a short precis of the recent history of his illness, for example:

S – *You were on the ward with us for 6 weeks, Jim, and I know that they were 6 very uncomfortable weeks with disturbed nights, lots of tablets, side-effects and endless needles. Your breathing was a bit better when you went home but now you're back in hospital again sooner than either of us expected. How are things today?*

- Involve the patient: note how the student has used an open question to invite facts or emotions. Good listening skills and handling Jim's emotional responses prepare for the most difficult part of the interview. It is good technique to paraphrase and summarise repeatedly:

S – *So, your breathing is so bad that you haven't had a wink of sleep since you went home and are wondering if it's all worthwhile.*

- Explain the dilemma:

S – *Someone with a heart condition as bad as yours may suddenly take a turn for the worst. In fact, the heart may stop beating. If that happens, there is no time to ask you what you would like us to do. If we were to restart your heart, we might prolong a situation which you find intolerable. We'd hate to do the wrong thing for you.*

- Ask a direct question: the discussion which leads up to the question may have to beat around the bush to bring Jim gently to the point of decision. However, he must be absolutely clear about the decision which is being made.

S – *If your heart stopped beating, would you want us to restart it for you?*

- Respond to any emotion or uncertainty, reach a decision or agree to defer it.

S – *I can see how distressing it is for you to face up to how ill you are. I can see that it's a hard decision for you, but you have said that life is so bad that you wouldn't want your heart to be restarted. Have I understood you correctly?*

Support and after-care

The danger of such a discussion is its apparent finality once a 'Do not resuscitate' order is agreed. In fact, the decision can relieve distress and offer hope by addressing the real needs of a terminally ill patient. These may include:

- Discussing the likelihood, imminence and mode of death
- Communication with other family members
- Promising support from doctors and nurses
- Agreeing treatments to relieve symptoms
- Attending to other practical issues, e.g. 'putting his affairs into order'.

Ending

As with all interviews, this one must be closed sensitively. For example:

S – *So, Jim, it sounds as though you weren't surprised by what I had to say. In fact, you're rather relieved to have talked about dying because you're very understandably afraid of it but haven't felt able to ask. You don't want us to call the cardiac arrest team if you collapse suddenly. We've agreed that I'll talk to your niece and that we won't rush to send you home again. Most important of all, Jane and I will make sure we're available to you to talk again. We'll work together to see if we can make those nights better. Do you have any other questions or are there any other things you'd like to say?*

Core skill: Discussing resuscitation status with a patient

1. Get the setting right.

2. Use appropriate verbal and non-verbal skills, and pace the discussion.

3. Set the scene with a narrative of the patient's illness.

4. Explain the need for a resuscitation decision.

5. Ask the question.

6. Respond, throughout, to the patient's emotions.

7. Discuss support and after-care.

8. Summarise and close.

SUGGESTIONS FOR FURTHER PRACTICE

If you have an opportunity to practise this skill with a simulated patient, take it. You could role-play the interview with a colleague, but be aware that emotionally loaded situations like this can be quite painful to simulate. Have decisions been made for the patients on your ward, and how fully were the patients involved in them? Perhaps you should tactfully bring this up on a ward round, and be sure to sit in on any interview that follows.

COMMUNICATION SKILLS

COMMUNICATION 3	**Teach inhaler technique**
Level:	*
Setting:	**An examiner and a healthy volunteer. Dummy pressurised aerosol inhaler provided**
Time:	**5 min**

TASK

E – *Tom has asthma. Please teach him how to take a dose of two puffs of this bronchodilator inhaler.*

RESPONSE

Your tasks are to explain clearly, rehearse the skill with the patient and test proficiency. The skill of giving a clear explanation is described in Communication 6: Explain 24-h urine collection; read that now and then go through in your mind or on paper the components of good inhaler technique.

Your response should include:

- Explain the way the bronchodilator works: by *relaxing the air passages in your lungs.*
- Explain the need for the bronchodilator solution:
  - To *reach as deep down into your lungs as possible.*
  - To *stay in your lungs long enough to be absorbed.*
- Demonstrate the procedure silently: *I am now going to show you how to use the inhaler.*
- Talk through the steps of the procedure:
  - Remove the mouthpiece cover.
  - Shake the canister.
  - Hold the inhaler vertically in your dominant hand with your index finger over the top and the mouthpiece close to your mouth.
  - Breath right out.
  - Put the mouthpiece *in your mouth with your lips tightly round it.*
  - Press firmly down on the body of the inhaler *as you start to breathe in.*
  - Take in a deep breath slowly so that the spray *goes deeply into your lungs.*
  - Hold the breath for 10 s.
  - Breathe out and, after a few moments, go through the whole process a second time.
- Ask the patient to perform the procedure.
- Correct errors and repeat until the skill has been mastered.
- Explain common problems:
  - Difficulty handling the inhaler (problems with manual dexterity).
  - Not triggering the spray at the right moment; typically too late.

- Not breathing the spray right down into the lungs.
- Not holding the spray in the lungs long enough for it to be absorbed.
- Invite questions, comments or concerns.
- Test understanding; e.g. *what do you feel are the important points in the explanation I have just given you?*

E – *If someone had difficulty activating the inhaler at the right moment, what alternative devices could you offer?*

- A device with a large volume chamber so that the patient can inhale after (rather than simultaneously with) activating the spray.
- An inhaler device that is triggered by breathing in.

E – *Please name some important educational points or common errors that you would emphasise when teaching patients about the use of inhalers for asthma. Do not confine yourself to this type of inhaler.*

- Beta$_2$ agonists and anti-cholinergics:
  - These rapidly control symptoms and can be taken as needed, within a specified dose range.
  - The recommended dose should not be exceeded. If it fails to control symptoms, the patient should contact a doctor.
- Inhaled steroids:
  - These only work if taken regularly. They are not effective if just taken during acute attacks.
  - Particularly in high dose, they can cause oral thrush. It is advisable to wash the mouth out after using them.
- Salmeterol and cromoglycate:
  - Like inhaled steroids, they must be taken regularly.

Core skill: Teaching a patient a procedure

1. Explain simply and clearly the purpose of the procedure.

2. Demonstrate the procedure silently.

3. Go through the steps of the procedure demonstrating and explaining them.

4. Ask the patient to perform the procedure.

5. Correct errors and ask the patient to repeat the procedure until they have mastered it.

6. Discuss common problems.

7. Test understanding, invite questions or comments.

8. Close.

COMMUNICATION SKILLS

SUGGESTIONS FOR FURTHER PRACTICE

Hospital wards are full of patients with poor inhaler technique. Ask a patient to demonstrate how they use their inhaler, and describe any difficulties they experience. Watch a patient being taught to use an inhaler and ask if you can do so yourself. Talk to a pharmacist about the finer details of bronchodilator therapy.

COMMUNICATION 4	**Discuss with a carer**
Level:	***
Setting:	You are seated opposite the examiner who 'vivas' you
Time:	10 min

TASK

E – *You are a house officer. Michael, a 34-year-old man with muscular dystrophy, has arrived in casualty with pneumonia. He is conscious but drowsy and does not respond when you ask him questions. The general practitioner sent a letter which states that he is normally mentally alert and recently completed an Open University Degree, but his physical condition has worsened progressively such that he is dependent on his parents for most aspects of his care. You are going to admit him to your ward. His father came to hospital with him. You meet him in the corridor. He asks how Michael is. How would you respond?*

RESPONSE

Insensitive handling of carers is a common cause of complaint; however, there is potential for ethical conflict because the doctor's primary responsibility is to the patient. The core skill box provides a framework for this type of discussion.

Core skill: Discussion with a carer

1. Introduce yourself.

2. Establish the carer's identity and relationship with the patient.

3. Use listening skills to:
   - Obtain factual information that the patient is not able to give you himself.
   - Show that you respect the carer's expertise.

4. Identify and acknowledge interdependence between the patient and carer.

5. Involve the carer as far as you can in making decisions, without compromising the autonomy of the patient (See Attitude 1: Giving information by telephone).

Introduce yourself

This entails much more than identifying yourself. You should invite Michael's father to sit down with you in a private place, and allow enough time for as full discussion as he would like. Use all the same inter-personal skills (described in the Introduction to this section, page 240) as you would use with a patient.

Establish the carer's identity

A chance encounter with a person in the corridor does not give you license to start divulging confidential information. You need to ask who you are speaking to. Exactly when you ask is a matter of judgement. Preface your question with an explanation (*I'm sure you will understand that, out of respect to Michael, I need to be sure who I am speaking to. May I ask you to say who you are?*). The relationship between a father and son is usually straightforward. Sometimes the carer is a common-law partner or neighbour. Under those circumstances, you must explore the relationship tactfully and make a judgement about the person's right to obtain information or influence treatment.

Use listening skills and identify and acknowledge interdependence between the patient and carer

Although you have a primary duty to the patient, you should use this interview with the father to clarify his role in Michael's care, acknowledge it and obtain whatever information you need to care for him. Michael is dependent on his parents. Hospitalisation can be a very difficult turn of events because it means that a carer who normally takes 24-h responsibility loses all sense of involvement and control. Michael's father is likely to understand him in a way that a health professional meeting him for the first time cannot. Therefore, he is an essential source of information if, as in Michael's case, the patient cannot give you factual information. Remember also that his father may be very close to and, in his own way, dependent upon Michael. Give him ample opportunity to ask questions, and use your skill as an empathic listener to identify and respond to the emotional content of his questions, and the thoughts that lie behind them. You may only be able to give provisional answers to questions at present.

E – *What specific information would you seek from Michael's father?*

The worst answer would be 'a full medical history'. Give a more focussed answer, concentrating on important points for a severely disabled patient with pneumonia. Think for a moment and come up with some headings in your mind, which could be:

The pneumonia
What previous respiratory illnesses has he had? Are there any symptoms to suggest that he aspirates when he swallows? Has he recently been in hospital or received antibiotics, as either of those situations would affect the choice of antibiotic therapy?

Functional status and quality of life
You should obtain a full description of his level of disability, dependence and quality of life. Drowsiness and unresponsiveness in a patient with muscular dystrophy and pneumonia spells respiratory failure. A decision may have to be made how aggressively he should be treated; to be specific, whether or not he

should be ventilated. An overall assessment of Michael's quality of life and prognosis is needed to inform that decision.

Michael's previously expressed wishes

Although mortally ill, John is a mentally competent adult whose rights are paramount. A crucial aspect of the discussion is to determine what treatment he would wish and whether he had made an 'advanced directive'; given his slowly deteriorating incurable disease and high level of intellectual attainment, he might well have done so.

E – *Michael's father tells you that he has not prepared an advanced directive, but has asked to be 'given a fighting chance' if he becomes severely ill. What actions would you take?*

- Measure blood gases; is he in respiratory failure?
- Perform basic investigations including a chest radiograph, biochemical screen, blood count and cultures of blood and sputum (if a specimen can be obtained)
- Consider antibiotic therapy; a junior doctor would be well advised to discuss that decision with a more senior colleague.
- Arrange chest suction if he has retained secretions.

SUGGESTIONS FOR FURTHER PRACTICE

Communication with carers is a major duty of house staff and it is one that can be shared by medical students. You should not conduct such important interviews as this one unattended but you can certainly 'go solo' in less grave situations. As you approach finals, you should ask a more experienced doctor if they will sit in while you speak to relatives or carers and give you constructive criticism of your technique

COMMUNICATION SKILLS

COMMUNICATION 5 Endoscopy

Level:	***
Setting:	**The examiner briefs you before asking you to interview a simulated patient**
Time:	**10 min**

TASK

E – *You are a house officer who has just returned from a week's leave. Mrs Taylor is a 50-year-old woman who was admitted with non-cardiac chest pain while you were away. The pain has settled and she is due to go home today. Your registrar rings you to say that she has a microcytic anaemia and needs an out-patient gastroscopy. Please speak to her about this. Call yourself 'Dr'.*

RESPONSE

A careless student could make a serious mistake here by relaying on to Mrs Taylor the registrar's instruction that she needs a gastroscopy, rather than *asking* her. This station is testing your knowledge of anaemia and gastroscopy, without which you cannot explain the situation to the patient. It is testing your ability to give the explanation clearly. Finally, it is testing your attitude. Failure to see the issue of informed consent in this situation would be marked harshly (see Communication 7: Lumbar puncture, for the core skill of obtaining consent). This dialogue illustrates how you might talk to Mrs Taylor:

S – *Good morning, Mrs Taylor. My name is Dr Proudfoot. I hope you will excuse me that I am unfamiliar with your case. I have just come back from holiday. My registrar tells me that you are better and ready to go home today.*

P – Yes, I'm right as rain. Can't wait to get out of here.

S – *That's understandable. There is one important test result I need to discuss with you. Your blood count shows that you are anaemic.*

P – I've been anaemic since I was a child. I told the GP but he wouldn't believe me. Said the blood test was normal; but my daughter could tell I was anaemic just looking at me.

S – *This time the blood test really <u>is</u> abnormal. You definitely are anaemic.*

P – Told the doctor, I did, years ago. He insisted that the test was normal.

S – *The blood test suggests that you could be losing blood from your stomach. That could also explain the pain that brought you into hospital. It is important to find out if there is something wrong with your stomach so that you can be given whatever treatment you need. My registrar has recommended that you should have a camera test to see if you are losing blood from your stomach.*

P – I'm not having one of those things stuck down my throat. You can forget that. I've been telling the doctor for years and he wouldn't listen. Been anaemic since I was a child and now you want to stick a camera down my throat. Forget it!

The student approached the request for consent quite appropriately but has met resistance. Gastroscopy is commonly described as a 'camera test' so the choice of words was reasonable.

It is likely that Mrs Taylor is resistant because she is afraid. It would be tempting to tackle this problem factually, and assume that any sensible patient will be persuaded by your logic, but that could easily turn this interview into a confrontation. Here is one way to avoid that:

S – *You're obviously not keen on having the test.*
P – You could say that.
S – *I would like to understand why the idea bothers you so much?*
P – How would you like to have a camera stuck down your throat?
S – *Are you concerned that it will be very uncomfortable?*
P – Yes; and you never know what they'll find if they go sticking things down your throat.
S – *You're concerned what the test may show?*
P – Concerned; that isn't the word.
S – *Could you tell me what you <u>do</u> feel about the test?*
P – More terrified than 'concerned'. There was this woman at work ... but I've been anaemic since I was a child so I don't need anyone sticking a camera down my throat.

This dialogue illustrates some of the cardinal principles discussed in the Introduction to Communication Skills:

- Discuss feelings before facts.
- Put feelings into words.
- Explore the reasoning that lies behind the feelings.

See Communication 9: Respond to a patient's dissatisfaction, and Communication 11: Respond to a patient's distress, for a fuller discussion of how to handle emotionally charged situations. The student responded appropriately and identified that the patient was using denial as a defence against fear. At this point, he continues to acknowledge Mrs Taylor's concern and tries to help her develop a more realistic understanding of the situation:

S – *What is it you're terrified of?*
P – The big C.
S – *It is understandable that talking about anaemia and having a camera test should terrify you. There is a small chance that you have a tumour in your stomach. It is far more likely that the explanation for your anaemia is a simple one like an ulcer or inflammation of the lining of your stomach which can be treated; or there may be nothing wrong with your stomach at all. By doing the camera test there is every chance that we will be able to put your mind at rest. Even if you have a tumour, the best thing is for it to be found as early as possible. If you do not have the test, we risk missing giving you treatment that could help you.*

COMMUNICATION SKILLS

P – Nip it in the bud, you mean. But like I said, I've been anaemic since I was a child.

S – *Do you know anyone who has had a camera test?*

P – No.

S – *Before the test, you would be given something to relax you. The test involves passing quite a thin tube through your mouth into your stomach. It is not particularly uncomfortable and you would remember little about it afterwards. You would only need to come up to the hospital as a day case and would be back to normal the next day.*

In this dialogue, the student has:

- Explained the consequences of having and not having the gastroscopy.
- Described the test in a way that is appropriate to this patient, concentrating on clear practical information and not giving unnecessary technicalities.

E – *Supposing Mrs Taylor flatly refused the endoscopy, what would you do?*

The answer could include:

- Ethics: a competent patient has the right to refuse treatment even if the doctor believes that the refusal is neither in their interests, nor reasonable.
- Communication: a doctor has a duty to demonstrate respect towards a patient, and maintain communication with them, even when they have made what the doctor regards as an unwise choice.
- Practical management: it would be sensible to explain the situation to Mrs Taylor's general practitioner (by telephone and/or in the discharge summary), and give her a follow-up appointment to allow her to reconsider her decision.

Core skill: Responding to resistant behaviour

1. Recognise that flippancy, non-communicativeness and evasive behaviour may be forms of resistance that need to be explored.

2. Explore the patient's point of view on the situation.

3. Acknowledge and show respect for any emotions shown by the patient.

4. Explore the reason(s) for those emotions.

5. Explore the patient's knowledge and perceptions of the situation.

6. If the patient is receptive, give them relevant information.

7. Help the patient balance the pros and cons of any proposed course of action so that they can make their choice.

8. Respect the patient's autonomy.

9. Remain polite at all times; avoid confrontation.

SUGGESTIONS FOR FURTHER PRACTICE

How often do the clinicians you work with inform patients adequately about planned investigations or treatments and how fully do they involve them in decisions? Do they always obtain informed verbal consent? Discussing the need for a procedure is a task that a student can perform under the supervision or on behalf of a doctor. Volunteer to do so and become experienced at it.

COMMUNICATION 6	**Explain 24 h urine collection**
Level:	*
Setting:	Interview with healthy volunteer
Time:	5 min

TASK

E – *Please explain to this person how to collect a 24 hour urine sample.*

RESPONSE

S – *Good morning (shakes hands), my name is Tom. Could you tell me your name?*
P – Anthony.
S – *I have been asked to explain to you how to collect a 24 hour urine sample. Is that OK with you?*
P – Yes.
S – *Have you ever collected one before?*
P – No.
S – *The aim is to collect every drop of urine you pass over a 24 hour period into this container. It is up to you to choose the most convenient time to do the collection. It doesn't matter when you start but many people find first thing in the morning the best time. Go to the toilet, spend a penny and flush it away as normal. From then onwards, every time you pass water, do so directly into this container, or use a clean dry jug and pour it carefully into the container. The important thing is to catch every drop of urine. Is my explanation clear so far?*
P – Yes.
S – *The last time you should pass urine into the jug is <u>exactly</u> 24 hours after the start, but of course this time the urine goes into the jug, not down the loo. Please deliver the container to the hospital within at most 24 hours of finishing the collection. Does that seem clear?*
P – Yes.
S – *Do you have any questions?*
P – No.
S – *Could you repeat my explanation back to me?*

P repeats explanation

S – *Yes, it's really a question of getting every drop of urine into the container over a period of exactly 24 hours and then returning the container to the hospital the same day. Where people go wrong is by making an incomplete collection, perhaps because they forget once or twice, or by making the collection shorter than 24 hours. Thank you for listening so carefully to my explanation. I hope you won't find it too much trouble. Goodbye (shake hands).*

E – *Suppose the patient was being investigated for hypertension, what might you want to measure in a 24 hour urine and what preservative would need to be in the container?*

This station has two main components; the COMMUNICATION SKILL of giving an effective explanation (for which most marks will be awarded), and KNOWLEDGE of the investigation of hypertension/renal disease.

Core skill: How to give an effective explanation

1. Sit where you and the patient can easily see each others' faces at the right distance apart.

2. Introduce yourself and establish the patient's identity.

3. Identify the task.

4. Obtain approval to proceed.

5. Establish the patient's prior experience.

6. Give a clear explanation without jargon and make appropriate use of colloquial language.

7. Pace the explanation appropriately, including pauses.

8. Check the patient's understanding, by asking him to repeat the information back to you.

9. Summarise.

10. Close.

11. Show respect and courtesy throughout.

Knowledge of 24 h urine collection

Hypertension may be 'essential' (no underlying cause) or 'secondary' to endocrine or renal disease. Essential hypertension may cause proteinuria and renal impairment. Table 7.1 shows some of the indications for 24 h urine collection in a hypertensive patient, and the details of sample collection.

SUGGESTIONS FOR FURTHER PRACTICE

This station will make it very clear how much 'nuts and bolts' experience you have acquired, and how practically aware and competent you are. If you do not know how patients should do simple procedures like 24 h urine collections, you need to take a more practical interest in day-to-day medicine. Everyday clinical experience gives you ample opportunities to practice the very important

COMMUNICATION SKILLS

Table 7.1 Indications for a 24 h urine collection

Diagnosis	Relationship with hypertension	Measurement	Sample collection
Renal impairment	May cause it or be a consequence of it	Protein excretion, creatinine clearance	Container with no preservative
Phaeochromocytoma	Causes it	Urinary catecholamine and metanephrine excretion	Urine container should contain acid preservative
Cushing's disease	Causes it	Urinary free cortisol excretion	Container with no preservative
Primary aldosteronism (Conn's syndrome)	Causes it	May measure 24 h potassium excretion	Container with no preservative

communication skill of explaining simple procedures. Try applying the learning points above to:

- giving an insulin injection
- using a bronchodilator inhaler (then see Communication 3: Teach inhaler technique)
- measuring peak flow.

COMMUNICATION 7	**Lumbar puncture**
Level:	**
Setting:	Interview with standardised patient
Time:	5 min

TASK

E – *Mrs Taylor is a 43-year-old housewife who has been admitted to hospital as an emergency with headache. The consultant has found neck stiffness and is concerned that, although she is not seriously ill, she might have meningitis. He wishes her to have a lumbar puncture. Please obtain verbal consent from her to perform the lumbar puncture.*

RESPONSE

There are four components to this station:

1. Communication
2. Ethics
3. Knowledge of meningitis
4. Knowledge of lumbar puncture.

(Data 4: Cerebrospinal fluid, discusses the interpretation of lumbar puncture results.)

Communication

Communication 6: Explain 24 h urine collection, has described in detail how to explain a procedure to a patient. This station demands many of the same skills but is explicitly testing your knowledge of informed consent; you must use your communication with the patient to demonstrate your awareness of the ethical/legal issues without being prompted.

Ethics

Before performing the procedure, you have an ethical and legal obligation to obtain *informed* consent. This means that you must explain:

- Why the procedure must be done and any possible alternatives.
- The nature of the procedure and any significant risks or discomfort associated with it.

You must *ask* for permission to do the test. It is unethical to frame your question in a way that makes it hard for the patient to say no.

COMMUNICATION SKILLS

265

Why the procedure must be done

Because:

- Meningitis is potentially serious.
- The most serious forms of meningitis can be effectively treated with antibiotics.
- Delay in making the diagnosis and starting treatment worsens the outlook.
- Lumbar puncture is the only way of excluding meningitis.
- While it is possible to give an antibiotic without performing a lumbar puncture, there is less chance of making an accurate diagnosis and that would create serious difficulties if Mrs Taylor did not respond to the antibiotic.

Nature of the procedure and risks

Your explanation should include:

- The need to lie still, curled up at the edge of a soft mattress for up to half an hour.
- Cleaning the skin with cold antiseptic solution.
- The local anaesthetic ('freezing the skin') which may sting for a moment or two.
- A possible sensation of pressure when the needle is introduced.
- A possibility that the person doing the test may put their hands round the patient's neck momentarily (Queckenstedt's manoeuvre) or ask the patient to take some breaths in and out.
- A possibility of a sudden, sharp tingle in one or other leg.
- The likelihood of an ache in the patient's back and a headache after the procedure.

Core skill: Obtaining informed consent

1. Introduce yourself and establish the patient's identity.

2. Identify the task.

3. Explain:
   - Why the procedure must be done
   - Possible alternatives
   - The nature of the procedure
   - Risks and discomforts associated with it.

4. Ask permission, using an open-ended, non-directive question.

5. Show respect for the patient's autonomy; do not behave coercively.

6. Invite the patient to ask any further questions.

7. Close.

- The possibility of the patient being confined to bed for a time after the procedure.

E – *How could you minimise the discomfort of Mrs Taylor's lumbar puncture?*

If you have not mentioned the comfortable bed and local anaesthetic, you must do so now; however, it would be pointless to repeat it if you have already said it. It is possible to minimise headache after lumbar puncture by using a finer-gauge needle, and one with a blunt rather than a cutting tip. If patients develop headache after lumbar puncture, injecting venous blood into the lumbar puncture site ('blood patch') can reduce headache (Serpell et al, 1998). There is little evidence that keeping the patient lying down for 24 h helps at all.

SUGGESTIONS FOR FURTHER PRACTICE

If you have never seen a lumbar puncture, you must do so. They are performed daily on neurology wards. If you cultivate a good relationship with the medical staff, you may be allowed to do one but first you must learn the indications and the technical details of the procedure. Practise interpreting CSF results (Data 4).

REFERENCE

Serpell MG, Haldane GJ, Jamieson DRS, Carson D 1998 Prevention of headache after lumbar puncture: questionnaire survey of neurologists and neurosurgeons in United Kingdom. Br Med J 316: 1709–1710

COMMUNICATION SKILLS

COMMUNICATION 8	**Break bad news**
Level:	***
Setting:	An examiner and standardised patient
Time:	10 min

TASK

E – *Please imagine yourself to be a General Practitioner; use your own surname and call yourself Doctor. Your next patient is Mr Michael Dent. You do not know him personally but the notes tell you that he consulted your partner recently with weight loss which Mr Dent put down to work stress, although your partner picked up on night sweats as a possible clue to something more sinister. Various tests were done, one of which was a full blood count. The report states: Marked neutrophilia with some myeloid precursors, moderate anaemia and thrombocytosis. Probable chronic granulocytic (myeloid) leukaemia. Needs urgent referral for bone marrow examination. Mr Dent has come for the result of the test. Please call him in and give him the result of the test.*

RESPONSE

There are two components to this station: The skill of breaking bad news and your knowledge of chronic granulocytic leukaemia. It is primarily a test of your skill as a communicator but you cannot handle the situation unless you know enough about the disease to answer the patient's questions and the examiner will undoubtedly award some marks for knowledge.

Breaking bad news

This can be broken down into the following steps.

The setting and your behaviour

- Position
- Eye contact
- Body language
- Your listening skills
- Opening the interview in a way that builds trust
- Pacing the interview well and 'having time'
- Allowing the patient to have the appropriate degree of 'control'.

Invite Mr Dent into the room, introduce yourself, offer him a chair and seat yourself across the corner of the desk reasonably close to him where you can make good eye contact. Use a fairly neutral opener such as: *I believe you saw my partner a couple of weeks ago because you had lost some weight and have come today for the results of your tests.* Listen attentively to and encourage any response. Pick up on any emotional content in what Mr Dent says or any personal details that seem important to him.

Exploring the patient's perception of their condition and prepare them

- Get Mr Dent as involved throughout by always **asking before telling**.

You could both explore his perceptions of his condition and prepare him for bad news by asking a question such as: *I believe you put your loss of weight down to all the stress you have been under at work. Did you think of any other possibilities?* Now the skill is to encourage him to respond and elaborate. You can do this by using non-verbal skills (silence, a posture which conveys interest in what he says, nodding in agreement) and verbal skills (echoing important components of what he has said, inviting him to say more, simple words like 'yes', 'hmm', 'and then' and putting his emotions into words: *so you were worried about that possibility*).

Finding out what the patient wishes to know

Handled well, this is another way of preparing the patient for the bad news to come and gives you all-important information about how much detail you should go into today. You might ask: *Are you the sort of person who likes to know all about his medical condition?* Or: *If there were an abnormal test result, how much would you want to know about it?* Again, concentrate hard on developing your relationship with him and learning how best to meet his needs.

Giving information

- Build up the bad news layer by layer.
- Give information as kindly as possibly and in small pieces.
- Avoid jargon and use the patient's own words whenever possible.
- Allow time for the patient to respond.
- Check understanding.
- Give realistic information about outcome and treatment options.
- Leave room for hope.

A good approach in this case would be to go through recent events as a narrative, building up the result of the blood report and the actions that can be taken. For example: *You saw my partner 2 weeks ago because of the weight loss which you put down to work stress. He was concerned by the sweating attacks you had been experiencing and arranged blood tests to check if there was any serious cause for them. Your blood count is not completely normal. You are anaemic and have some abnormalities in some of the other cells in your blood. I know that I am using many technical terms. I'd like to check what they mean to you.* Another question which encourages patients to respond is: *Does all this make any sense to you?*

Patients' responses are so individual that you cannot predict what will happen next. Your main goal will be to agree a hospital referral with Mr Dent and much information may have to be left for future conversations with yourself or a haematologist. Information which may be covered includes:

- That he probably has a serious blood disorder

COMMUNICATION SKILLS

- That it may be chronic granulocytic leukaemia
- That a bone marrow examination is needed to confirm the diagnosis
- That treatment is possible.

There may be a host of other questions. Your skill is to allow those which are immediately important to Mr Dent to come to the surface and answer them as best you can.

Acknowledge and respond to the patient's emotions

- Non-verbally
- Practically; e.g. by offering tissues
- By putting emotions into words and saying that they are understandable ('legitimising' them)
- By exploring what lies behind that emotion.

Hand-in-hand with transmission of information goes the task of handling Mr Dent's emotional response. This is likely to be very strong when the word 'leukaemia' is used. The sensitive practitioner will weave backwards and forwards between the two tasks: *It obviously hurt you a lot to ask how long you are likely to live. It would help me understand how you are feeling if you could explain why you asked that question. I will give you the most honest answer I can.* Common responses to bad news are anger and denial. Try to analyse how Mr Dent is responding. If he doesn't show any emotional response, invite one with the question: *How does this news make you feel?* Encourage him by asking (more than once, if necessary) if he has any other concerns or questions.

Planning and ending

- Summarise facts and emotions
- State the ways in which you can help:
  - Referral

Core skill: Breaking bad news

1. Get the setting right.

2. Use good verbal and non-verbal skills; allow as much time as needed.

3. Explore the patient's perceptions of their condition and prepare them.

4. Find out what the patient wishes to know.

5. Give information in plain language and at an appropriate pace.

6. Acknowledge and respond to the patient's emotions.

7. Make a plan.

8. Summarise and draw the interview to a close.

COMMUNICATION SKILLS

  - Treatment
  - Palliation
  - Meeting/telling other family members.
- Make concrete offers of help (which you can and will fulfil)
- Conclude the interview by agreeing on next steps
- Invite questions and give another opportunity to express concerns
- Be prepared to give more time and re-run parts of the interview.

SUGGESTIONS FOR FURTHER PRACTICE

You are unlikely to be given the task of breaking bad news as a medical student but you must make sure that you sit in when others do so. You should consider the times you've been given unwelcome news. How did you react? How did the other person handle it? How would you have liked them to handle it differently? Finally, ask patients with serious problems how they were told, how they responded and how they would like you to handle the task. Communication 13 describes another application of the 'breaking bad news' approach.

COMMUNICATION 9	**Respond to a patient's dissatisfaction**
Level:	***
Setting:	The examiner briefs you before asking you to interview a simulated patient
Time:	10 min

TASK

E – *As a senior student, you are shadowing the house officer on your ward. He goes off sick and you are asked to carry his bleep. Mr Noble, a 63-year-old patient recently admitted to the ward, has asked to speak to a doctor. You look at his notes and see that the cause of admission is fast atrial fibrillation. He was diagnosed thyrotoxic a year ago. He received carbimazole for 9 months which was then stopped and he has had no further treatment. The doctor who admitted him is in little doubt that his thyrotoxicosis has relapsed and is the cause of the atrial fibrillation. Please interview Mr Noble.*

RESPONSE

S – *Good morning Mr Noble. My name is Paul. I am a final year medical student. Dr Cartwright, the house officer, is unwell and I'm covering him. You wanted to speak to a member of the medical team. How can I help?*

P – That Doctor Singh or whatever his name was, the one who took all my details in casualty, he said that it was stopping the thyroid tablets that's landed me here. That's not right if you ask me. It's all well and good him saying that. It's obvious that I've not been treated right and it's you lot that's to blame. I want to speak to the top man.

OSCEs are anxiety-provoking enough without having to face this sort of situation. Perhaps your examiners would never put you on the spot like this, but the reality of medical life is that you may have to respond to difficult challenges even when you are feeling tired or otherwise vulnerable. This situation tests:

- How you act under pressure
- Your attitudes
- Your communication skills
- Your knowledge.

Apart from feeling that this is an unfair exam, you are likely to be flustered by the tone of Mr Noble's voice and unsure of your knowledge of thyroid disease and its treatment. Whether as a student, a house officer or in an OSCE exam your options include:

- Asking someone more senior to take over.
- Regarding his view as a factual misconception and correcting him.

- Recognising the tone of anger in his voice and trying to take control of the situation by being firm.
- Taking his anger on yourself and becoming angry, guilty or anxious.
- Responding constructively to his emotions.

The skilled professional will:

- Recognise the emotional content of this problem.
- Follow two simple rules of communication skills (and of 'patient-centred practice'): handle emotions first, then facts … and … ask before telling.
- Use a repertoire of skills appropriate to handling anger.
- Use any knowledge he has to enlighten the discussion.

It would be an abdication of professional responsibility to terminate the interview at this point, even for a medical student. Handled correctly, Mr Noble's mind may be put at ease. Handled incorrectly, Paul may create a confrontation or dig a deep hole for himself by overreliance on factual knowledge.

Responding to anger

There are two important points which underpin effective communication with an angry person:

- It is usually secondary to another emotion such as fear, guilt or uncertainty. Finding the primary emotion will achieve a better outcome than taking the anger purely at face value.
- Minor disagreement can explode unpredictably into a showdown. The dialogue should, from the start, work towards de-escalation and resolution.

There are many similarities between the handling of anger and the handling of anxiety (Communication 5), distress (Communication 11) and bad news (Communications 8 and 13). No matter how flustered or angry you feel, try to behave calmly.

Non-verbal aspects
Attend to the patient's and your own comfort and need for privacy. If possible, sit at the same level and at an appropriate distance. Position yourself so that you can easily make eye contact. Do not lean threateningly towards the patient. Avoid dismissive or defensive gestures (e.g. slouching back with arms folded). Do not fidget or move unnecessarily but show that you are listening. Use eye contact to communicate interest and concern but don't glare.

Verbal aspects
The patient should be allowed to feel in control of the interview and given every encouragement to express his views. Allow him plenty of opportunity to say what he has to say, with verbal encouragement to show that you are listening. Speak calmly and slowly. Do not raise your voice.

Dialogue
Following the guidelines above, Paul might respond to Mr Noble's initial demand as follows:

COMMUNICATION SKILLS

S – *So you feel angry about the way you have been treated and feel it is to blame for how you are now.*

P – Too right I do. You go to the doctor to be put right, not to be messed up so that you land up in hospital.

S – *You feel that your treatment has been messed up?*

P – I certainly do.

S – *It is understandable that you should feel that way and question your treatment if you end up in hospital.*

P – Then you're gasping for breath, having ECGs and wondering what surprise they've got in store for you next.

S – *It sounds as though you're feeling really bad.*

Paul is working entirely at the emotional level, encouraging Mr Noble to vent his feelings. Now he is beginning to obtain information, but still responding with concern. He might now explore the source of the anger.

S – *Anyone who's been through what you've been through might feel dissatisfied about their treatment but I'd like to understand what has upset you most of all.*

P – Never had a day's illness in my life until they started treatment for that thyroid trouble. Now I'm having heart tests, heart drugs and the full works.

S – *Are you worried about your heart?*

P – Well wouldn't you be?

Paul has now begun to define the cause of the anger and is well on the way to defusing it. He has handled the interview well without (yet) needing any knowledge of thyroid disease; nor has he made any judgement about the rights and wrongs of Mr Noble's treatment. The communication skills he has used are:

- Reflection of emotion
- Paraphrasing
- Empathising and giving legitimacy to the patient's feelings
- Finding out how the patient sees the facts of the case
- Avoiding disagreement.

At this point, it would be wise for him to check if Mr Noble still wishes to speak to someone more senior. The direction of the discussion suggests that he may not.

Achieving resolution

As the interview proceeds, the interviewer will attempt to:

- Steer it away from the point of conflict (i.e. the fact that the carbimazole was stopped).
- Avoid any comments which might unjustifiably incriminate others.
- Identify constructive actions that he, the patient and others can take (i.e. control the atrial fibrillation and hyperthyroidism).
- Give clear and accurate information, or undertake to seek it.
- Find any realistic grounds for optimism in the face of anxiety, uncertainty etc.

COMMUNICATION SKILLS

The facts of this case

The examiner might ask you about the management and prognosis of hyper-thyroidism and/or atrial fibrillation.

Overall, only about 25% of patients achieve a lasting remission of hyper-thyroidism, even after prolonged antithyroid drug therapy. The chance of remission falls with age so one might argue that Mr Noble should have had radio-iodine treatment; nevertheless, his management was typical of UK practice. If there was a management error, it was that his thyroid function was not checked sooner after carbimazole was stopped. Perhaps Mr Noble was asked to have a blood test and did not do so; perhaps he is blaming the medical profession so stridently because he feels guilty about a failing of his own. Assuming a thyroid function test confirms hyperthyroidism, he is likely to be re-treated with carbimazole and referred for radio-iodine therapy once it is controlled. If his hyperthyroidism turns out to be relatively mild, some endocrinologists would give radio-iodine without carbimazole pre-treatment.

Unpleasant though it is, the prognosis of fast atrial fibrillation may be very good. Mr Noble is likely to be heparinised (to prevent embolism), digitalised and treated for any heart failure. Atrial fibrillation of short duration with a treatable underlying cause may revert to sinus rhythm spontaneously. Urgent cardioversion would be indicated for fast atrial fibrillation with haemodynamic compromise. Cardioversion may actually precipitate embolism from the fibrillating atrium so it should be deferred until he has been anticoagulated for 2 weeks or so if at all possible. That also allows time for spontaneous reversion to sinus rhythm.

Core skill: Responding to anger

1. Get the setting right.
2. Use good verbal and non-verbal skills.
3. 'Reflect' the patient's anger by putting it into words.
4. Give legitimacy to the patient's feelings without incriminating others.
5. Achieve a clear understanding of the patient's perspective.
6. Steer the discussion away from the point of conflict.
7. Find common ground, build on it and attempt to achieve resolution.
8. Avoid confrontation at all costs.

SUGGESTIONS FOR FURTHER PRACTICE

Sadly, life is all too full of opportunities to practise handling anger in partners, friends, colleagues and complete strangers. Seek out a dissatisfied patient on your ward and explore the source of their dissatisfaction. Although described in a medical context here, the skill of handling anger is a 'life skill'. In the heat of a row with your nearest and dearest, see if you can step outside the situation, see it for what it is, de-escalate it and resolve it. Both home life and professional practice may benefit!

COMMUNICATION 10	**Cross-cultural communication**
Level:	***
Setting:	Structured oral examination
Time:	15 min

TASK

E – *A thin Asian man of 68 attends the health centre, where you see him in an emergency surgery. The receptionist tells you that he speaks no English but is accompanied by his son who is acting as interpreter. The son tells you that his father is passing too much water. What do you think the cause might be?*

RESPONSE

History 10: Thirst and polyuria, lists some causes of polyuria. Up to one in ten Asian men over the age of 60 have diabetes mellitus so that must be your first suggestion. Phrase your answer in a way that shows your awareness of the importance of this disease in Asian people.

E – *The practice computer shows that he has been diabetic for 10 years and is treated with Metformin 850 mg tds and Gliclazide 160 mg bd. He was offered insulin treatment but flatly refused it. The practice nurse did a finger-prick glucose measurement before he came in to you; it is 25 mmol/l. Why do you think he might be presenting with polyuria now?*

Poor glycaemic control in a patient with type 2 diabetes may be due to:

- 'Secondary failure' of oral hypoglycaemic therapy; in other words, the pancreas has failed, tablets are no longer working and insulin is needed.
- Over-eating.
- Not taking the prescribed medication.
- Intercurrent illness; for example, urinary infection which increases insulin resistance and makes the normal treatment less effective.

This scenario has been constructed around an Asian patient. You would demonstrate awareness of the influence of cultural factors on disease if you included factors specific to Asian people in your answer. During Ramadan, Muslim patients may not eat anything (including their tablets) during daylight hours, and often eat a single large meal after sunset. This often causes loss of diabetic control. In addition, Asian patients may have beliefs about the cause of illness and the effectiveness of treatments that differ from the conventional Western view. Complementary therapies are often used (sometimes as well as, sometimes instead of, conventional therapy), particularly a bitter vegetable called 'Karela' which has only weak glucose-lowering properties and is wide' available.

E – *In this case, you are going to communicate with the patient through an interpreter. How would you set about doing that?*

Do not assume that the patient cannot understand you

Although your primary communication may have to be with the interpreter, watch the patient carefully. If he shows signs of understanding and responding to what you say, see if you can strike up any direct communication, no matter how limited.

Communicate with both the interpreter and the patient

When you are speaking to the interpreter, use all your normal communication skills, including eye contact. During the dialogue between the interpreter and the patient, direct your attention to the patient, and use your non-verbal communication skills both to develop the relationship and interpret how they are responding. At times, you may add emphasis to what you are saying by looking at the patient when you speak, even if your words need subsequently to be interpreted.

Communicate simply and in small 'chunks', to avoid overloading the interpreter

Look out for any evidence of the hazards of using an interpreter

- Your words, and the patient's response, may not be transmitted faithfully.
- The interpreter may not understand technical words.
- The patient, or interpreter, may shy away from delicate subjects.
- The interpreter may dominate or control the patient.

Core skill: Communicating through an interpreter

1. Make no assumptions; find out what the patient can and cannot understand.

2. Address both the patient and the interpreter.

3. Communicate simply and in small 'chunks'.

4. Be aware of the dangers of using interpreters:
   - Incorrect transmission or misunderstanding of information
   - Avoidance of delicate topics
   - Domination of the patient by the interpreter.

E – *It is Ramadan. Please describe how you would explore whether that could be affecting his glycaemic control.*

The text that follows gives a framework for cross-cultural communication and applies it to this case.

Explore and clarify the problem

Explain to the patient that his diabetes has become poorly controlled, and ask him why he thinks this has happened. Ask him directly about his eating and tablet taking, and any other factors (e.g. inter-current illness) that might have affected his control. You will get the best information by asking him to describe his habits over, for example, the last 2 days, rather than asking broad general questions about compliance.

Clarify the cultural dimension

Ask him whether there is anything special about his culture or religion that might be affecting him.

Show acceptance of the cultural dimension

People from some cultures may see health professionals as powerful and judgemental. A comment such as: *Ramadan must be a very difficult time for someone like you who has a strong religious faith but also has an illness which needs regular treatment* will bring you and the patient closer together in finding a solution to the problem.

Identify the patient's explanatory framework

If, for example, a patient sees diabetes as a judgement from God on him as a sinner, rather than a widely prevalent disease in which the beta cells fail, he will logically choose 'non-compliance' rather than tablet-taking during Ramadan. By exploring his attribution of the illness, and contrasting it with your own, you may succeed in finding common ground. You may also find out more about his self-care, such as reliance on folk healers.

Clarify the view of the individual within his cultural norm

There is a grave danger of stereotyping in cross-cultural communication. Each individual Muslim person has their own view of Ramadan, which will determine whether a conflict of religion versus medical need can be resolved. You could ask an exploratory question such as: *Do you feel there are any circumstances when the fast can be broken, for example if it puts someone's life in danger?*

Explain the situation

In this case, the patient is experiencing polyuria and feeling ill because he is caught between religious observance and medical need. It is his responsibility to choose a course of action but it is yours to put him in the position to do so, by laying out the facts. For example: *You are a strict Muslim and the fact that you have diabetes has made you feel it is all the more important that you observe Ramadan strictly,*

COMMUNICATION SKILLS

but this means that you are not having essential treatment. You are feeling ill and you may even be in some danger as a result.

Explore solutions and involve other agencies

In this case, the patient has refused insulin so his only hope of feeling better is a more satisfactory balance of diet and tablet-taking. His son is acting as interpreter and is party to the discussion. He may help the patient choose what is in his interests, and enlist help to resolve any religious conflict.

Core skill: Cross-cultural communication

1. Be aware of, identify and show acceptance of the cultural dimension of illness.

2. Work within the patient's framework of understanding.

3. Explore the patient's view within the norms of their culture.

4. Explain, as far as possible within the patient's terms of reference.

5. Explore solutions and involve other agencies.

SUGGESTIONS FOR FURTHER PRACTICE

Build confidence in cross-cultural communication through the ethnic minority patients you meet. You could learn, through them, such things as:

- Naming conventions, and the correct way of addressing people.
- Family and social structures. How autonomous are people, or are they strongly bound into family, social or religious norms?
- Dietary customs.
- Observance of religions.

COMMUNICATION SKILLS

Respond to a patient's distress

Level:	**
Setting:	A 'real' patient and an examiner observing
Time:	20 min

TASK

You have been given 20 minutes to take a history from a 'real' patient. The examiner is sitting inconspicuously in a corner with a clipboard. The interview has not gone well. Your patient is a 65-year-old lady weighing 18 stone who gives indirect and wordy answers to your questions. Ten minutes into the interview, you have established that she has pain in both hips but has been turned down for hip surgery until she loses 3 stone in weight. She has talked a lot about the poor bus service to the village in which she lives and the distance from her cottage to the bus stop. You have found it difficult to structure the interview – it isn't even clear to you what her presenting complaint is. You are beginning to panic because you have only 10 minutes to go and haven't got beyond the 'presenting complaint'. Now, tears well up in her eyes and she says 'Oh dear, oh dear, oh dear'.

RESPONSE

This is the stuff of nightmares but it happens in clinical practice and could happen in an examination. There are two people – you and the patient – in deep distress! Faced with calamity, it is human nature to struggle to retain control and that is how students (and doctors) usually respond. Your best bet is to stay calm and look calamity in the eye. For you to 'take control' is the wrong tactic because the situation is completely beyond your control. The patient's distress is the overwhelming consideration and has to be acknowledged. Only by getting that right will you restart any productive dialogue.

Responding to distress

How to handle emotionally charged situations is discussed in Communications 8, 9 and 13 as well as the core skill box.

In practical terms, you could start handling this situation by:

- Saying to her: *I can see that you are very upset.*
- Finding tissues and offering her one.
- Giving her your undivided attention, perhaps with a sympathetic smile, eye contact and silence.
- Drawing closer to her; perhaps by leaning towards her. You may judge that you should put a friendly hand on her arm.

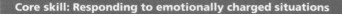

> **Core skill: Responding to emotionally charged situations**
>
> 1. Do not run away from strong emotion; it will not go away.
>
> 2. Help the patient feel in control of the interview.
>
> 3. Deal with emotions before facts; put the emotions into words and offer them back to the patient.
>
> 4. Seek to understand the emotions. Be clear what the patient is feeling and identify the source of those feelings.
>
> 5. Show your empathy verbally and non-verbally.
>
> 6. When the time is right, encourage the patient to elaborate on the background to her emotions.

(Communication 9: Respond to a patient's dissatisfaction, provides a detailed dialogue for a situation that has many features in common with this one.)

Getting the interview back on the rails

Your choice is between regarding the display of emotion as an unwelcome interruption and returning to your previous questioning strategy, or building on the new understanding that you and the patient have established. The latter is the better strategy because:

- The interview was already going very badly. The outburst has told you that your patient's level of emotional distress is too high for your previous history-taking approach to work. Your only hope of continuing the interview fruitfully is to continue acknowledging the emotional problem and keep the patient in control by working within her frame of reference.
- If you can move away from a strictly 'disease-focussed' interview, you stand a better chance of finishing your fast-disappearing 20 minutes with a meaningful assessment.

You have actually obtained some pathological information:

- Osteoarthrosis needing hip replacement.
- Obesity as a potential anaesthetic complication.

As a skilled and responsive interviewer, you have now added to this an understanding of the emotional dimension of the problem, very likely a feeling of desperation and frustration about:

- Being disabled by pain and immobility.
- Inability to lose the amount of weight demanded by the hip surgeon.

You could build on this by considering the functional effects of the illness. Now that you have the patient's full cooperation, the information about the cottage

COMMUNICATION SKILLS

and the bus service could be revisited to build up a precise picture of the impact of the illness on her activities of daily living. Now that she has 'unloaded emotional baggage' and found that you understand her, you may find her a responsive and helpful interviewee.

You could explore the patient's ideas, concerns and expectations about the illness. A statement about her obesity being 'due to her glands' could be regarded as an irrelevant throw-away, or an indication that she attributes obesity to factors outside her control and will not adhere to any diet.

Having gained her confidence by working within her terms of reference, she may be much more cooperative when you ask her the normal questions of the medical interview. Any remaining time can be used to ask questions that are relevant to the medical problems you have uncovered.

HOW DO I KNOW HOW I AM DOING IN AN EXAM?

The short answer is not even to try to judge because you will get it wrong. Students misread the responses of their examiners as often as they get them right. They emerge from an exam convinced they have failed because the examiner asked hard questions (usually a sign that they have done OK). They are flabbergasted when they fail because 'the examiner was so pleasant' (actually giving them every shred of encouragement as they plough themselves). It would be a daft examination system that failed the student in this scenario because she left some gaps in her history. The only way she would plough the exam would be to struggle on to take a full history rather than make the best of an unwelcome situation. An examiner observing an interview should give credit for:

- The communication skills exhibited.
- The student's adaptability to the responses and expressed needs of the patient she is interviewing.
- The quality of the assessment of the patient, including biomedical and psychosocial aspects.

Skilful handling of the patient's distress and adaptability to an unexpected situation should attract high marks.

SUGGESTIONS FOR FURTHER PRACTICE

Most of us shy away from emotionally charged situations. However, there has been plentiful research showing that patients are most satisfied with doctors who not only respond to, but give precedence to the emotional component of their problem. Next time you interview a patient, see what emotional content you can identify and pay particular attention to it. If you develop a good rapport, you may ask the patient to critique the way you responded. As with handling anger (Communication 9), you can blur the boundary between your professional and private life and use the same skills in your dealings with your partner, friends or colleagues.

COMMUNICATION SKILLS

COMMUNICATION 12 | Discuss HIV testing

Level:	***
Setting:	A volunteer student role-playing a young male patient
Time:	10 min

TASK

E – *You are attached to a GUM clinic. Jim is 23 and has asked for an 'AIDS test'; the task of discussing this with him has been delegated to you. Please discuss the test with him before the blood is taken.*

RESPONSE

This is an example of HIV testing for the 'worried well'. The test must not be performed unless the issues have been carefully discussed, the grounds for doing it have been established and the patient's informed (verbal) consent obtained. You may find it helpful to go through this station in conjunction with History 6: Erectile dysfunction, which discusses another facet of communication about sexuality. The examiner will be observing your:

- Communication skills with an anxious patient on a sensitive topic.
- Awareness of the ethical issues surrounding HIV testing.
- Knowledge of HIV and AIDS.
- Skill as an educator.

The core skill box sets out the framework of the discussion, explained more fully in the paragraphs that follow it.

Core skill: Discussion in preparation for an HIV test

1. Introductions and guarantee of confidentiality.

2. Assessment of risk.

3. Discussion of HIV/AIDS.

4. Discussion of the test.

5. Discussion of legal, financial and social implications of the test.

6. Discussion of consequences of positive and negative test.

7. Request for consent.

8. Advice about behaviour pending test result.

Introductions

Introduce yourself, including your role. Establish the patient's identity, and use the introductions to build rapport.

Guarantee confidentiality

Tell the patient that the discussion you are about to have and the result of the test, if done, will be handled with complete confidentiality.

Assess risk

You should introduce this part of the interview with an open question such as: *Why are you considering having this test?* Use listening skills, as described in Communication 8: Break bad news, to help the patient explain their concerns. Relevant points to cover are the patient's:

- Current state of health, including any pointers to HIV/AIDS.
- Sexual orientation.
- Sexual behaviour, including numbers of partners, type of intercourse (vaginal, anal – penetrative, receptive), use of condoms.
- Partners: promiscuity and sexual orientation.
- History of sexually transmitted disease.
- Country of origin, travel and sexual behaviour while overseas.
- History of drug abuse.
- History of blood or blood product transfusion, or organ donation.

At this stage, you should give the patient a rough estimate of risk (low, medium or high).

Discuss HIV/AIDS

Check the patient's knowledge of the disease and give them some basic information about:

- The fact that you can test for HIV infection, not for AIDS (the term 'AIDS test' is a misnomer).
- The window period between infection and seroconversion (normally no more than 3 months) during which a false negative result may be obtained.
- Transmission, primary HIV infection, seroconversion, the asymptomatic period when lymphocyte counts decline, then AIDS.

If the patient is seeking the test because of very recent unprotected intercourse and is likely to be in the window period, they may opt to defer the test. They must be encouraged to practice safe sex in the meantime.

Discuss the test

- Check that the patient now understands that the test is for HIV antibodies.

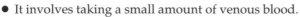

- It involves taking a small amount of venous blood.
- Tell the patient when the result will be available.
- Tell the patient that the result will be given verbally, ideally by you (since you are the one who has reached agreement with them to do the test).

Discuss the legal, financial and social implications of the test

- When applying for a mortgage, insurance etc., the patient may be asked whether they have had an HIV test (other than a mandatory insurance test) and may be refused insurance if they admit to it.
- If the test is positive, the patient will be strongly encouraged to give consent for his GP and dentist to be notified and the result will then be permanently in his GP records.
- The patient may be asked about his HIV status at employment medicals, although they are not legally obliged to divulge information.
- If positive, the patient's partner(s) should be informed.

Consequences

You should assess the patient's ability to cope with the implications of a positive test, and prepare them for it. You are assessing their personal readiness, and support mechanisms. Some implications of a positive test are:

- It would need to be repeated to confirm its positivity.
- It would give the patient greater certainty, albeit of an unpleasant nature.
- The patient would be offered continuing medical support and follow-up.
- It would allow early treatment, including anti-retroviral treatment and prophylaxis against opportunistic infections.
- It would allow the patient to alert others (partners, health professionals) of the risk of transmission.
- It would motivate the patient to practise safe sex, safe drug use etc.

If negative:

- The possibility of a false negative has to be considered.
- It would give the patient reassurance.
- The patient should still behave responsibly to minimise their risk of HIV infection.

Obtain consent

Having already estimated and discussed the risk, the patient should now be encouraged to weigh up the pros and cons of having the test done and asked for their decision.

Advice about behaviour pending the test result

The patient should be particularly careful to practice safe sex, safe drug use etc. until the result is known.

E – *Supposing the test came back positive, he refused to tell his partner and you knew he was practicing unsafe sex. Would you tell the partner?*

Ethical issues surrounding confidentiality

The UK General Medical Council has published guidance to doctors in its booklet 'HIV and AIDS: the ethical considerations'. It tells doctors that, in those circumstances, they should try very hard to persuade the patient to tell his partner. If he still refuses, 'the doctor may consider it a duty to seek to ensure that any sexual partner is informed, in order to safeguard such persons from infection'. The booklet stresses that any doctor who breaches confidentiality will need to 'be prepared to justify' this action.

SUGGESTIONS FOR FURTHER PRACTICE

Originally, only trained AIDS counsellors were allowed to conduct the pre-test discussion. Increasingly, it is being seen as a mainstream clinical skill. As a house officer, you may have to obtain the permission of an ill patient to have the test when no counsellor is available. You should attend a GUM clinic and observe the procedures surrounding AIDS testing, and the implications of a positive result.

COMMUNICATION SKILLS

COMMUNICATION 13 | Give information to a patient

Level:	***
Setting:	The examiner meets you in the office of the ward where the exam is taking place and briefs you before taking you to the bedside where you find a 60-year-old female simulated patient sitting on the edge of her bed. You conduct an interview with her
Time:	10 min

TASK

E – *You are the duty house physician on call over the weekend. You are asked by the nursing staff to see Mrs Wells who wants to talk to a doctor. Her notes tell you that she was admitted on Friday night with a GP referral letter stating that she has been investigated at another hospital and found to have extensive adenocarcinoma from an unknown primary. Her admission is for pain control. A chest X-ray done on admission confirms the appearance of metastases but the notes are otherwise uninformative. It is clear that the admitting team literally admitted her and then went off for the weekend. Please interview her. I will observe you.*

RESPONSE

Here you are confronted with a difficult situation that is not uncommon in the life of a house officer. It is difficult both because of the seriousness of the patient's condition and because you are tackling it in the face of uncertainty about:

- The patient and her reactions to the situation
- The diagnosis
- What she already knows
- The facts (for example, how long she is likely to live).

The 'breaking bad news' framework (see core skill box in Communication 8: Break bad news) is the one to use here. When breaking bad news, it is good practice always to ask before telling. That will help you find out what Mrs Wells knows, her perceptions of the situation, her concerns and her needs. You may well be able to strike up a good relationship by doing so. You may not be able to answer all her questions, but you can agree a strategy to find as good answers as possible in the near future. You can work out a plan to support her through this illness. This discussion uses the framework from the Breaking bad news core skill box.

The setting and your behaviour

The side of a bed in an open ward is not ideal for private and emotionally loaded conversations but you must make the most of it. Pull the curtains round, speak in a low voice, position yourself and Mrs Wells to create an atmosphere of intimacy and use the other skills described in Communication 8.

Explore the patient's perception of their condition and prepare them

You do not know what she knows so you may find that you are giving bad news for the first time. Alternatively you may be answering specific questions from a well-informed patient. Either way, a suitable opener might be: *What have you been told about your condition?* You must then use the techniques described in Communication 8 to draw out from Mrs Wells as much of her factual grasp of the situation, her perceptions and emotional reactions as you can.

Find out what the patient wishes to know

This is made easier by the fact that Mrs Wells has asked to speak to you. You could introduce this part of the interview with a question such as: *What was in your mind when you asked to speak to a doctor?* Throughout this part of the interview you are drawing Mrs Wells out by:

- Non-verbal communication: showing concern and interest.
- Verbal communication: responding to what she says in a way which encourages her to say more.
- Acknowledging the emotional content of what she says: *I can see that it is upsetting for you to ask that question.*

Give information

Communication 8 reminds you of the techniques of giving information. Your starting point is Mrs Wells' perceptions of her disease and your assessment of what she wishes to know. Possible concerns are:

- The seriousness of her disease
- How long she has to live
  - A patient with extensive adenocarcinoma is unlikely to live as long as a year.
- Whether her disease can be controlled and what treatments she will receive
  - There is probably no treatment which will even slow the disease but you can offer her realistic hope by discussing palliative treatments.
- The possibility of controlling her pain
  - That should certainly be possible; you should discuss ways of monitoring her pain relief.
- What other symptoms she may experience
- How the disease is affecting other family members and what information they have been or should be given
- How long she needs to stay in hospital.

You will feel vulnerable handling this situation because you share the patient's uncertainty about many of these things. However, your shared uncertainty can help you develop a sense of partnership with her if you handle the remaining stages of the interview well. Be aware that there is a limit to how much she can take in. Do not overload her with information.

Acknowledge and respond to the patient's emotions

The patient may not be seeking factual information at all but may want to vent emotions. Certainly, she will be *experiencing* emotions. Communication 8 suggests how you may respond to them.

Planning and ending

The OSCE examiner may be particularly interested in how you handle this part of the interview because it tests the basic competence and knowledge to be expected of a house officer. The plan that you agree with the patient may include:

- Monitoring pain control and adjusting treatment
- Liaising with the team who will look after her during the week
- Obtaining notes from the other hospital, test results etc. and discussing them with Mrs Wells to reduce her uncertainty
- Meeting other family members
- Involving other support services such as a MacMillan nurse or social worker
- The timing of her discharge
- Making yourself available to speak to her again.

SUGGESTIONS FOR FURTHER PRACTICE

You should involve yourself in the management of patients with incurable disease during your clerkships, observe their care and speak to them about their experiences. In particular, practise the skill of responding to their emotions. If you have the chance of practising this skill in role-play or with a simulated patient, seize it.

COMMUNICATION SKILLS

CHAPTER 8

Attitudes

Introduction

Traditional medical examinations examine the knowledge of students in great detail. Final examinations also always included an assessment of a student's ability to take a history and perform a clinical examination (but not other types of clinical skills). In contrast, the attitudes of graduating students have never been formally assessed, yet attitudes link very closely to professional behaviour and are a major cause of complaint from patients.

Prompted by the General Medical Council, many schools are starting to include assessments of attitudes within the formal (pass/fail) examinations. In an OSCE, this will take the form of a structured oral, in which an examiner will describe a difficult situation and then ask you to discuss your analysis of the issues involved and how you might respond.

At these stations, the examiner will be potentially assessing you in a number of different areas:

- Do you know the medico-legal framework in which doctors work and can you apply your knowledge to the situation that the examiner has set out?
- What ethical principles do you think are important for a doctor and how would you apply these principles to the clinical situation described by the examiner?
- Are you aware of national guidelines? In the UK these are set out in the 'Duties of the Doctor' (GMC, UK) and other publications, for example on consent.

In addition to these ethical frameworks, the examiner will want to see how you will show empathy and understanding for the patient. (Look at the communication skills section of this book and try to act in their *not your* best interest.) You should also emphasise how you are working in a team and would always seek help and guidance when you feel that you are out of your depth. It is very important that you demonstrate that you would involve senior colleagues and consult with your indemnifying body (e.g. the Medical Defence Union or Medical Protection Society in the UK) and the GMC.

THE STATIONS

The content of this section falls into five main categories (some stations fall into more than one):

Confidentiality

- Criminal activity: Attitude 1
- A problem with epilepsy: Attitude 2
- Risk of infection: Attitude 4
- Giving information by telephone: Attitude 5
- Problems with your colleague: Attitude 6

Autonomy

- A difficult haematemesis: Attitude 3
- Giving information by telephone: Attitude 5
- A cry for help?: Attitude 7

Medico-legal

- Criminal activity: Attitude 1
- A problem with epilepsy: Attitude 2
- A cry for help?: Attitude 7
- Terminal care: Attitude 8

Duty to society

- Criminal activity: Attitude 1
- A problem with epilepsy: Attitude 2
- Risk of infection: Attitude 4
- Problems with your colleague: Attitude 6

Respect for life

- Terminal care: Attitude 8

HOW TO REVISE FOR ATTITUDINAL STATIONS

You should be aware of the nationally accepted ethical standards. In the UK these are laid down in the GMC guidance in 'Duties of a doctor'. There are also other GMC publications that you should read such as those dealing with issues as consent and infectious diseases. You will also find valuable, particularly in relation to medico-legal matters, the information given out by the indemnifying bodies, which, in the UK, are the Medical Defence Union and the Medical Protection Society.

In your revision, you should also read through some of the stations contained in the communication skill section such as:

- Consent: Communication 7
- Team working: Communication 2
- Resuscitation status: Communication 2
- House officer responsibilities: Communication 5
- HIV testing: Communication 12
- Cross-cultural issues: Communication 10
- Serious illness in a patient with incurable disease: Communication 4

You might also read through a number of the history-taking stations that deal with complex issues (e.g. History 6: Erectile dysfunction).

ATTITUDE 1	Criminal activity
Level:	***
Setting:	Structured viva with an examiner

TASK

E – *You are the house officer on-call for general medicine. You are called to see a patient who has been brought in by his friend because of an asthmatic attack. The friend left very quickly and did not leave his name. The police arrive very soon after this. They ask you to give them some information on the patient as they suspect he was involved in a car-crash whilst escaping from a robbery. They also want to take a blood specimen for alcohol level. What should you do?*

RESPONSE

There are several complex issues in this case. The Road Traffic Act of 1988 states that if a driver may have committed an offence under the Act, then the police can require anyone to divulge information that may lead to the identification of the driver. However, as a doctor, you are bound by a duty of confidentiality not to give any **clinical** information without the consent of the patient. On this basis, you can confirm the identity of the person and when they were brought into Casualty, but cannot tell the police officer anything about his medical condition, without first talking to the patient.

Under the same Act, you can refuse to obtain a blood or urine sample if you believe that it is clinically inappropriate. The grounds for refusal include psychiatric illness. In this case, you should talk to the patient about the arrival of the police, what they want to know and their request for a blood sample. If the patient wants to provide a sample and you think that it is not detrimental to his health, then you may go ahead.

E – *When you start to undress the patient, you find a blood-stained knife in his jacket pocket, he is also muttering 'I had to do it'. What action should you take?*

The finding of a knife does not change the principle of confidentiality in relation to clinical matters. You may choose to override this if you think that there is a significant risk of serious harm or death to someone. The **implication** is that this is to prevent something happening in the future, not to shed light on something that has already occurred.

Remember you are accountable for your actions to both the courts and the GMC. As with the other attitudinal stations, **always** consider contacting senior colleagues, your indemnifying body and/or the GMC. There is **always** help at hand, it is better to ask.

ATTITUDES

> **Core skill: Dealing with potentially criminal incidents**
>
> The key considerations are:
>
> 1. As a doctor, you are bound by a duty of confidentiality not to give any **clinical** information without the consent of the patient.
>
> 2. You can refuse permission to obtain a blood or urine sample if you believe that it is clinically inappropriate.
>
> 3. As a doctor, you are accountable for your actions to both the courts and the GMC.
>
> 4. The duty of confidentiality can be overridden if you believe there is a significant risk of serious harm or death to someone.

SUGGESTIONS FOR FURTHER PRACTICE

The Accident and Emergency Department is the commonest area in which situations are dealt with that have potential medico-legal implications. You should talk to the staff about how they deal with the police in such matters as driving with excess blood alcohol.

ATTITUDE 2	**A problem with epilepsy**
Level:	***
Setting:	Structured viva with an examiner

TASK

E – *You are a house officer in the general medical unit. One of your patients is a known 23-year-old salesman who has epilepsy. He has just started to fit again after being fit-free for 5 years. You stabilise him on a new drug treatment. He is now asking you about returning to work. What information would you want from him and how would you advise him?*

RESPONSE

This is a common legal and ethics problem encountered by house officers. You must be able to describe how you would talk to the patient and what would govern your responses and actions.

The first step is to find out what his job is and whether it entails driving. If so, the law is very clear:

1. A patient can drive (on or off drugs) when they have been free of fits for 12 months, providing they do not have continued high likelihood of seizures (e.g. a known brain tumour).
2. If he/she has purely nocturnal (sleep) seizures he/she can drive, providing this pattern has been established for 3 years.
3. If he/she holds a PSV or LGV licence, he/she can drive, providing he/she has been fit free for 10 years and has been off drugs for 10 years and has been examined by a specialist.
4. It is the **patient's** responsibility to inform the DVLC of any change in their health that **might** affect their ability to drive.

The examiner will probably expect you to know Nos 1 & 4, but if you are in doubt, state that you would find out the relevant facts before talking to the patient. Most probably you will have to do this if the patient holds a PSV or LGV licence. You should also tell the examiner that you would record the discussion with the patient, including what you have told him, in the case notes.

E – *You discover that he is a driver and you tell him about the law on this. He tells you that he cannot stop driving as he will lose his job. He says that he will ignore your advice and 'the fit was just a one-off when he had been on a binge'. What do you do now?*

You should make sure that the patient understands that his medical condition

affects his right to drive and explain the legal position. The patient is at fault if he refuses to contact the DVLC. The onus is on a driver to inform the centre if anything 'MAY affect their ability to drive'. It is then up to the DVLC to make the final decision, not the treating doctor. If the patient refuses to contact the DVLC, you can suggest a second opinion, but you must clearly tell the patient not to drive until then.

E – *Some weeks later, you see him in town driving his car. In his records, the consultant has recorded that he has given up his driving licence.*
What do you do now?

If the patient continues to drive despite reasonable effort to persuade them otherwise, your duty of confidentiality to them can be overridden by concerns for the significant risk to others. In this case, should the patient have a fit whilst driving on a motorway, the consequences could be the death(s) of somebody else. You can involve the patient's partner/relatives in making it clear to them that they cannot continue to drive. As a final resort, if the patient refuses to stop, you should inform them that you are going to inform the medical adviser on the DVLC (in confidence).

Once the DVLC have withdrawn the patient's licence, they cannot take any further action even if the patient continues to drive. You should consider informing the police. Ultimately, if the patient has an accident, you could be subject to a Civil Suite for damages if you have not carried out your responsibilities.

Core skill: Epilepsy and the law

1. Ask about driving and how this would affect the person's job.

2. Knowledge about the law in relation to epilepsy:
   - A patient can drive with a standard licence (on or off drugs) when they have been free of fits for 12 months, providing they do not have continued high likelihood of seizures.

3. Advise the patient about their responsibilities.

4. Record what you have discussed with the patient.

5. Suggest that the patient might want to talk to a more senior doctor or his GP about driving.

6. Suggest that you would talk to the consultant about seeing the patient driving.

7. Awareness that you have the right to inform the DVLC if you think that the patient is going to continue to drive despite careful consideration of the position.

ATTITUDES

In summary, the ethical/attitudinal areas in this station are:

- Respecting confidentiality
- Recognising the need to inform others when a patient refuses to take personal responsibility
- Recognising that failing to act may put others at risk
- Realising that a doctor's duty may involve doing something to which the patient has not consented.

SUGGESTIONS FOR FURTHER PRACTICE

When you are talking to a patient with epilepsy, ask them about what they know about the law relating to driving. You should also talk to the doctors you are working with about how they handle such incidents and other issues relating to a patient's ability to drive (e.g. following a stroke).

ATTITUDE 3　A difficult haematemesis

Level:	***
Setting:	Structured oral with examiner

TASK

E – *You are the house officer on call for medical emergencies. You are fast-bleeped to casualty. There you find a 53-year-old man who is semiconscious and has been vomiting copious amounts of blood. His blood pressure is unrecordable and his pulse barely palpable. The Casualty officer has inserted a large intravenous line and Group O negative blood has just arrived. The staff nurse tells you that they have been through his clothing as they have undressed him. His name is John Abott and he has a card stating that he is a Jehovah's Witness and must not be given blood. What do you do?*

RESPONSE

You should look at Procedure 8 for general discussion about blood transfusion. In the case here you are called on to make an immediate decision. It is very easy to reason that you should give the blood as the person cannot give informed consent and will die if you do not act. However, Jehovah's Witnesses carry cards stating that they must not be transfused as they believe that the Bible forbids them to spill blood or make use of it.

You should also indicate that you would try to check with relatives that the carrying of a card indicates that this is the patient's current wishes. It would **not** be acceptable (the examiner would fail you) to give the blood whilst the patient was unconscious and not inform the patient. The GMC expects doctors to tell the truth.

Some groups of Jehovah's Witnesses will allow autologous transfusion (blood from the patient, stored and given back at the time of need – such as elective surgery).

Core skill: Respect for autonomy

1. As a doctor, you must respect a person's right to autonomy (self-determination).

2. This means that you must accept that a patient can refuse consent even if it appears to you to be irrational and is against your judgement.

3. Your acceptance of autonomy may mean that the patient may die.

ATTITUDES

Some groups will accept infusion of other fluids, so in this case (unless the card indicates otherwise), you could discuss with the examiner the use of plasma expanders.

SUGGESTIONS FOR FURTHER PRACTICE

You should arrange a session with the blood transfusion service and talk to them about what arrangements they make for patients who will not accept blood from someone else, but will have an autologous transfusion or other fluids.

It would also be helpful to talk to anaesthetists and surgeons about how they manage patients who are Jehovah's Witnesses.

ATTITUDE 4	**Risk of infection**
Level:	***
Setting:	Structured oral with examiner
Time:	5 min

TASK

E – *You are the house officer on a cardiology ward. A 55-year-old woman has been admitted under your care for cardiac catheterisation. She tells you that she is hepatitis B positive, but instructs you not to speak to anyone else about it, including the cardiologist. She is very firm about it. How do you react?*

RESPONSE

In this station, the examiner is looking for your

- Ability to analyse the problem
- Medical knowledge relating to the situation
- Ability to apply your medical knowledge
- Plan to incorporate action within an ethical framework that is in keeping with the 'Duties of a Doctor' (GMC, UK).

The first step is to talk at length with the patient about the difficulties that her condition is likely to pose for the health care team. As part of this discussion, you would explore why she has told you, but then stipulates that you must not pass your knowledge on to anyone else. If you can get her to express her feelings, there will probably be links to previous events and emotions.

If at the end of talking to her, she still refuses to allow you to disclose her hepatitis status to anyone else, her confidentiality must be respected. However, in this case, you may consider that failure to inform anyone else will place others at serious risk. It is then possible to breach confidentiality on a 'need to know' basis (e.g. the cardiologist performing the catheterisation), but the GMC (UK) state that these circumstances will only arise rarely and the doctor must be able to justify their action. You should always inform the patient about what you propose to do.

It would not be acceptable to agree not to tell anyone about the patient's condition or, as the other extreme, inform the patient that you must break confidentiality without any discussion around it.

In summary, the main attitudinal/ethical aspects are:

- The conflict between maintaining patient confidentiality and applying the principle of 'need to know' to confidential information.
- The legal obligations on a doctor.

> **Core skill: Handling information concerning risk to others**
>
> You should:
>
> 1. Discuss with the patient the reasons they do not want to disclose the information (but has told you).
>
> 2. Include in your discussion with the patient the potential risk for the healthcare team.
>
> If the patient still refused to agree to disclose their status, you should:
>
> 3. Inform the patient that the risk to others meant that you would have to talk to the relevant members of the team on a strictly 'need to know' basis.

SUGGESTIONS FOR FURTHER PRACTICE:

The risk of infection to others arises most often in relation to:

- Hepatitis B
- HIV.

You should arrange to spend time with the team looking after patients with HIV and observe how they counsel patients about testing for infection. You could also talk to the staff on renal units to determine how they handle the potential risk from Hepatitis B infection.

ATTITUDE 5   Giving information by telephone

Level:	***
Setting:	Structured oral

TASK

E – *You are a house physician on an elderly care unit. One of your patients (Edward Bruce) is an 89-year-old man who you admitted yesterday following a TIA from which he has made a rapid recovery.*

You know that Mr Bruce has previously been well and living independently on his own. You have just seen Mr Bruce and he is well and looking forward to going home.

In the ward office, you are asked by the ward clerk to speak to Mr Bruce's daughter. The person asks you 'what is the matter with my father'? How would you answer this?

RESPONSE

The first part of this station is concerned with confidentiality. All medical oaths from Hippocrates onwards have stressed this as the cornerstone of good clinical practice. The consequences of breaching confidentiality can be serious:

- Loss of trust by the patient
- Disciplinary action by the NHS
- Serious professional misconduct charge from the GMC
- Civil suit.

Table 8.1 illustrates the important considerations (constructs) in this case and describes good (mediocre and bad!) practice. A key communication skill involves talking to people (patients, carers, doctors, other professions etc.) over the phone. It is relatively easy to set up such OSCE stations and you should be prepared to play a role set for you by the examiner. The same principles apply as described in the communication section in this book.

In the first part of the case the key elements are:

- Checking who the person is.

On the telephone, check the identity of callers who request medical information by ringing them back. If you are sending a fax, make sure the machine receiving faxes is secure before sending patient details. You might also indicate to the examiners that many cases in which confidentiality is breached arise by over-hearing a conversation. You should make an effort to seek privacy.

Table 8.1 Confidentiality and right to self-determination. The following is a specimen rating guide used by examiners. You need to judge which category you would fall into

	Establishes caller's identity	Willingness to give information to caller	Willingness to withold information from patient	Discussion of autonomy/ confidentiality	Communication
Good	If in doubt over identity, suggests that he/she takes number and phone back	Explains to daughter why he/she cannot give information without patient's permission	Explains that cannot agree not to discuss medical problems with father	Explains that would not force information on patient, but would discuss as much as patient wanted to know	Suggests that discussion on the phone is not best and offers to speak to her if she comes into hospital / Explores why the daughter feels this way
Adequate	Asks who he/she is speaking to on the phone, but then accepts response	Informs daughter that cannot give information to her, but no clear explanation or discussion of reasons	Informs daughter that cannot agree not to discuss medical problems with father, but little explanation of why	Some ability to discuss patient autonomy and confidentiality	Superficial discussion of how might talk to patient about medical problems
Poor	Does not ascertain who the person is to whom he/she is speaking	Student gives out information to caller without hesitation	Readily agrees not to disclose information to patient	No consideration of self-determination or confidentiality	No consideration of communication skills involved

ATTITUDES

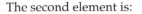

The second element is:

● Confidentiality.

Information held by the medical practitioner about a patient is confidential and must not be disclosed without the patient's permission (see also Attitudes 2 and 4). In this case, you should combine declining to talk the daughter about her father's medical problems with the communication skill of conveying the right of her father to confidentiality.

E – *The daughter says 'My father is a worrier, please do not tell him anything about his condition without telling me first so that I can decide what is best'. How would you respond?*

The key element (construct) is patient autonomy. Look at Table 8.1 and also Attitudes 7 and 8 for further discussion. Adults have the right to determine what they want to know, and do not want to know, about their illness. You should not allow yourself to be drawn into a contract with the daughter setting limits on your duties as the medical practitioner to her father. Again, this needs to be combined with the communication skill of discussing autonomy.

SUGGESTIONS FOR FURTHER PRACTICE

Observe how the medical staff you are working with (e.g. house officer, general practitioner, consultant) handle requests for information. Ask them to talk to you about the examples you have observed.

ATTITUDES

ATTITUDE 6	**Problems with your colleague**
Level:	***
Setting:	Structured viva with an examiner

TASK

E – *You are a house officer on a general medical unit. One night when you are on duty with another house officer, you notice that he appears to be acting strangely. He is quite dishevelled and his pupils are very constricted. What would you do?*

RESPONSE

Every doctor carries a responsibility to take all the necessary steps to protect the patients' interests. This has been emphasised recently by the GMC in relation to sick or poorly performing doctors. Once you have concerns about one of your colleagues, you have a duty not only to them, but also to their patients to do something. You cannot ignore the problem or suggest that it is the responsibility of the clinical tutor or someone else.

The first step is to speak to the house officer about your concerns and try to find out if there is anything wrong. You should do this by saying 'There is something that is bothering me and I need to talk to you about it. Can we go somewhere private?' If the house-officer says that there was nothing wrong, you would have to firmly say that you cannot accept that and that you would have to talk with someone more senior. Nor can you accept that it is just a 'little problem' or that you would not do anything unless 'it got worse'.

E – *You discover that he is abusing drugs intravenously, but he asks you not to tell anybody. What do you do now?*

Your overriding duty as a doctor is to report to the appropriate authority someone whom you *think* represents a risk to patients. This should take place even if confidentiality has to be broken. Failure to do so may amount to serious professional misconduct.

You should explain this to your colleague and that they have a responsibility to seek help. It is good practice to suggest that you would be willing to go with them. The following are appropriate people to talk to:

- Your colleague's educational supervisor
- The postgraduate (clinical) tutor
- Your educational supervisor.

You have to ensure that your colleague has sought help. If not, you have a clear responsibility to talk to someone about your concerns.

Core skill: Health of your colleagues

The elements of good practice are:

1. Explaining to house officer that you realise something is wrong and invite them to talk about it.

2. Explaining to house officer about duties to patients.

3. Explaining to house officer that they have a duty to seek help and if they will not do so, then you would have to talk to an appropriate person (postgraduate tutor, educational supervisor).

4. Offering to go with them to seek help.

SUGGESTIONS FOR FURTHER PRACTICE

You need to have read the relevant GMC publications which guide the ethics of medical practice in the UK:

- The Duties of a Doctor
- The New Doctor (covering the pre-registration house officer year).

ATTITUDE 7 | A cry for help?'

Level:	***
Setting:	Structured oral with examiner

TASK

E – *You are the house officer on-call for medical emergencies. A 79-year-old woman is brought into the Casualty department by her neighbour. She says that she does not want to stay. The neighbour says that the patient took a bottle of aspirin tablets 3 hours ago. The patient says that she wants to die. What would you do now?*

RESPONSE

In the first part of this station, there are three elements:

1. The patient wants to leave hospital.
2. The patient may have taken a serious overdose of tablets.
3. The patient is expressing a wish to die.

Your first action should be to try to persuade the patient to stay and talk to you about what has happened and, if possible, get her to consent to physical examination. You will then be in a better position to judge the seriousness of the overdose of tablets. You should also take the opportunity to corroborate your assessment with the account from the patient's neighbour. It is possible that the patient may deliberately mislead you on what she has taken (and how much) so that she achieves her aim of dying. Within this you also need to assess whether she has a psychiatric illness, particularly significant depression.

By coming to hospital with the neighbour, it is likely that, given sympathetic care, she will accept assessment, investigation and treatment. Patients can often be persuaded to comply with treatment by relatives, friends and nursing staff.

E – *You discover that she has no evidence of cognitive impairment and is not psychotic. However, she is adamant that she does not want any treatment and wants to die. Can she be treated against her will?*

A competent adult has the right to refuse treatment even if others, including doctors, believe that the refusal is neither in their best interests, nor reasonable. In this case, what matters is your assessment of whether the patient has the competency to give consent at the time of the proposed treatment. So, if you think that the patient has the capacity – treatment cannot be given. The key aspects of competency to give, or refuse consent are:

1. The patient's ability to comprehend and retain information.

2. Believe that information.
3. Weigh the information in the balance to arrive at a choice.

An irrational decision in itself does not compromise competency, it is the process by which the patient arrives at their decision, rather than the decision itself, which is the crucial factor in determining competency. If the test of competency is met, then the right of the patient to self-determination takes priority in law over the duty of care that you feel obliged to give.

It is good medical practice to obtain advice of more senior colleagues when faced with such a difficult scenario and also to record detailed accounts of circumstances and conversations. You also need to take into account whether competency is impaired through coexisting illness (e.g. dementia), drugs or alcohol. The more serious the potential threat to life, the greater the capacity required by the patient to make that decision.

E – *The son arrives in the department. He says that his mother has been depressed and suicidal since the death of his father 4 months ago. She has been on medication. He had been discussing with his mother's GP whether they could get a pyschiatrist to 'section her'. Does this change what you would do?*

Even without the son's intervention, you would probably want to involve a psychiatrist to assess the patient's mental state, including mood. It is possible to detain the patient under the 1983 Mental Health Act if she is suffering from a mental disorder (depression in her case) that means:

1. She is at risk of causing harm to herself or others.
2. The nature of the mental disorder means that she has to be treated in hospital.

If she is detained under the Act (Section 2 or 3), then you are allowed to give necessary treatment under Section 63

Core skill: Competency

In determining whether a patient has the capacity either to give, or withold, consent, you must judge if:

1. The patient can understand and retain information on the treatment proposed, its indications, and its main benefits as well as possible risks and the consequences of non-treatment.

2. The patient believes the information to be truthful.

3. The patient can weigh up the information in order to arrive at a conclusion.

Where there is any doubt – obtain the help of a more senior colleague.

ATTITUDES

SUGGESTIONS FOR FURTHER PRACTICE

There are two areas that the need to test competency to give consent commonly arise:

● Accident & Emergency department
● In-patient psychiatric units.

You should arrange to spend time observing how consent in such circumstances is dealt with and talk to the staff involved.

Terminal care

Level:	***
Setting:	Structured oral with an examiner

TASK

E – *It is 2:00 A.M. One of your patients on the ward is John Abbas, who has advanced metastatic prostatic cancer. He is fully aware of the diagnosis. He has been in great pain for a few days and most treatment options have been tried. He is now semiconscious, but very distressed. He is already on very large doses of morphine. His wife is with him and is very upset. She asks you to increase his dose of morphine to get rid of his pain. You know that his breathing is already poor and more morphine may cause a respiratory arrest. What do you do?*

RESPONSE

This is a situation that you may well have to handle as a house officer and will recur as you become more senior. A key aspect of this case is your communication skills in helping his wife. In your discussion, you should emphasise that your first duty is to your patient. You should also make it clear to the examiner that you empathise with how Mr Abbas's wife is feeling and that you would spend time talking to her about the situation, what has been done, and making it clear to her that you will do your best to relieve Mr Abbas's suffering.

You need to talk to his wife about the likely consequences of giving a larger dose of morphine. You would anticipate that it would help his pain, but, because of his poor respiratory state, it may cause a respiratory arrest and hasten his death. However, you should stress that your concern is to relieve the pain and that you are just explaining the other effects of narcotics.

In managing Mr Abbass's distress, the two principles you should be aware of are:

- Foreseeing is not necessarily the same as intending.
  If you intend to do something, then your aim will be to make this happen. This is not the same when you foresee that something might come about, but you do not set out to make it occur.
- The doctrine of double effect.
  'Double effect' is where you set out to relieve the pain and suffering of a patient despite foreseeing that the life of a patient may be shortened. This has been tested in Law and held to be permissible and in keeping with the duties of a doctor.

Core skill: Managing dying patients

The two principles for dealing with very ill patients with pain are:

1. Foreseeing is not necessarily the same as intending.

2. The doctrine of double effect.

SUGGESTIONS FOR FURTHER PRACTICE

In most hospitals, there are palliative care teams with hospital-based MacMillan nurses. You should arrange to spend an afternoon or a whole day with them observing how they manage patients and their carers. You should also take any opportunity to visit a hospice to gain more experience.

ATTITUDES

NORMAL VALUES FOR HAEMATOLOGY

Index	Range	Unit
White blood cell	4.0–11.0	$\times 10^9/l$
Neutrophils	2.0–7.5	$\times 10^9/l$
Lymphocytes	1.5–4.0	$\times 10^9/l$
Eosinophils	0.04–0.4	$\times 10^9/l$
Red blood cells – male	4.5–6.5	$\times 10^{12}/l$
Red blood cells – female	3.8–5.8	$\times 10^{12}/l$
Haemoglobin – male	13.0–17.0	g/dl
Haemaglobin – female	11.6–16.5	g/dl
Packed cell volume (male) (PCV)	0.40–0.54	l/l
Packed cell volume (female) (PCV)	0.37–0.49	l/l
Mean cell volume (MCV)	80.0–97.0	fl
Mean cell haemoglobin (MCH)	27.0–32.0	pg
Mean cell haemoglobin concentration (MCHC)	31.0–35.0	
Red cell distribution width (RDW)	11.5–15.0	g/dl
Platelets	150–400	$\times 10^9/l$
ESR – male	< 5	mm/h
ESR – female	< 7	mm/h
Plasma viscosity	1.50–1.72	cp
Reticulocytes	0.2–2.0	%
Serum B12	160–600	ng/l
Serum folate	2.0–10.0	µg/l
Red cell folate	125–600	µg/l
Ferritin – males	20–300	µg/l
Ferritin – female	12–250	µg/l – premenopausal
Ferritin – female	20–300	µg/l – postmenopausal
HbA2	1.8–3.5	%
HbF	0.2–1.0	%
G6PD	4.6–13.5	IU/gHb
Prothrombin time (PT)	12.0–16.0	sec
Activated partial thromboplastin time (APTT)	21.0–27.5	sec
Fibrinogen		
Fibrin degradation products	2.0–4.0	g/l
(D-dimer)	< 0.5	mg/l
Bleeding time (adults)	1.6–8.0	min

NORMAL REFERENCE RANGES FOR BIOCHEMISTRY

Index	Range	Value
Sodium	132–144	mmol/l
Potassium	3.5–5.0	mmol/l
Chloride	95–108	mmol/l
Bicarbonate	24–30	mmol/l
Urea	2.7–7.5	mmol/l
Creatinine	50–120	μmol/l
Glucose (fasting)	3.2–6.0	mmol/l
Glucose (random)	3.3–9.2	mmol/l
Bilirubin	1–20	μmol/l
Calcium	2.10–2.65	mmol/l
Phosphate	0.70–1.40	mmol/l
Total protein	60–80	g/l
Albumin	33–49	g/l
Globulin	21–38	g/l
Urate (female)	< 0.38	mmol/l
Urate (male)	< 0.42	mmol/l

Blood gases:

pH	7.38–7.42	
PCO_2	34–45 (4.5–6.0)	mmHg (KPa)
PO_2	90–100 (12–14.7)	mmHG (KPa)
Base excess	−2 to +2	

Enzymes:

ALP (adult)	25–110	IU/l
Amylase	10–87	IU/l
AST	5–45	IU/l
ALT (female)	5–45	IU/l
ALT (male)	5–45	IU/l
GGT	< 65	IU/l
CK	< 150	IU/l
LDH	200–500	IU/l

Cerebrospinal fluid:

Protein	0.25–0.75	g/l
Glucose (depends on blood sugar)	2.5–5.5	mmol/l

Hormones:

Thyroxine (T4)	50–150	nmol/l
Tri-iodothyronine (T3)	1.1–2.8	nmol/l
TSH	0.5–5.0	mU/l
Cortisol	200–650	nmol/l (07:00–09:00h)
	60–250	nmol/l (22:00–24:00h)
Urine free cortisol	< 300	nmol/24h

Lipids:

Total cholesterol satisfactory	< 5.2	mmol/l
Borderline	5.2–6.5	mmol/l
Unsatisfactory	> 6.5	mmol/l
Fasting triglycerides	0.3–2.0	mmol/l
Iron	12–30	μmol/l
Total iron binding capacity (TIBC)	45–70	μmol/l

Index